DR. WEINBERG'S GUIDE

to the

Best Health

Resources

on the Web

DR. WEINBERG'S GUIDE

to the ❧

Best Health

Resources
on the Web

❧

HARLAN R. WEINBERG, MD, FCCP

Collins

an imprint of HarperCollins*Publishers*

A special thank you to Carol Triplett for her spectacular technical assistance.
Many thanks to John K. Weinberg, MD, my brother, for his professional review.

Dr. Weinberg's Guide to the Best Health Resources on the Web is only a guide to
assist with clinical and educational information resources and does not substitute
for professional medical evaluation and treatment options for a specific
patient's medical illnesses. The author and publisher are not responsible or
liable for any damage or loss resulting from any medical evaluations, recommendations or treatments, nor for any of the information provided by the listed
websites. Always consult with your medical professional for individual patient
evaluation, treatment, and recommendations. All website addresses were accurate
and active at the time of publication. Use an Internet search engine to locate a
website if the published URL does not work. These links are only provided for
the user's convenience.

HarperCollins books may be purchased for educational, business, or sales
promotional use. For information, please write: Special Markets Department,
HarperCollins Publishers, 10 East 53rd Street, New York, NY 10022.

We would appreciate your input on medical websites for inclusion in our guide.
Please email your suggestions to internetmed@harpercollins.com.

First Edition

ISBN 978-0-06-137336-7

08 09 10 11 12 13 WBC/RRD 10 9 8 7 6 5 4 3 2 1

To my wife, Meryl, for everything.

To my daughters, Jaime and Victoria,
for their love and inspiration.

FRANKFORD

In memory of Dana and Christopher Reeve,
for whom there were no insurmountable obstacles.

CONTENTS ∽

Contents

Contents

INTRODUCTION ✎

M y fellow professional colleagues and patients worldwide, wel-
come to my *Guide to the Best Health Information on the Web*. I
have compiled this book after practicing medicine for twenty years,
specializing in pulmonary disease. I am also the director of the medical intensive care unit of Northern Westchester Hospital in Mt. Kisco,
New York, a post I have held for the past five years.

The rapid growth of medical information on the Internet has cre-
ated a complex maze of health-reference materials. Patients and
health care professionals alike are faced with the problem of information overload and need a means of choosing current, reliable, and
academically sound resources. The formidable goal of this book is to
provide for you access to the best professional health-care resources
available on the Internet. This educational reference guide will elim-
inate the need to search thousands of sites and will help focus your
medical search, improving your efficiency in selecting the most ap-
propriate medical information.

How to Use This Book

Let me simplify what can be a very difficult task for even the experi-
enced medical Internet user. First, the selection process may begin
with the "General Health Resources" chapter, a valuable starting
point. The sites listed in this first chapter cover a very broad range of

health topics. Review these websites to help determine a general over-view of your health education needs. Then, you will want to review a health topic by selecting individual website resources that are listed under specific clinical topics in the Table of Contents. Please remember that these medical searches will require you to invest your time, but they will make you a more informed patient, caregiver, or health professional.

The selection of websites in this book should not be your only source of health care information. Always remember that a consultation with your own physician(s) should precede any medical decision making or treatment recommendations.

Your health care is the most important concern for *medical professionals focusing on* patient safety and *improved* outcome. *Continuing* education, empowerment and active participation will make *a* difference in receiving or *providing* health care.

—HARLAN R. WEINBERG, MD, FCCP

General Health Resources ∽

Search these databases for all clinical topics

Up to Date
www.uptodateonline.com

Expansive clinical information covering Adult Primary Care and
Internal Medicine, Allergy and Immunology, Cardiology, Endocri-
nology and Diabetes, Family Medicine, Gastroenterology and
Hepatology, Hematology, Infectious Diseases, Nephrology and
Hypertension, Neurology, Obstetrics-Gynecology OB/GYN and
Women's Health, Oncology, Pediatrics, Pulmonary and Critical Care
Medicine, and Rheumatology.

Subscription required only for access to professional content.

eMedicine
www.emedicine.com

Expansive clinical information covering Clinical Procedures,
Dermatology, Emergency Medicine, Hand Surgery, Internal
Medicine, Neurology, Orthopedic Surgery, Ophthalmology,
Otolaryngology and Facial Plastic Surgery, Plastic Surgery,
Pediatrics, Physical Medicine and Rehabilitation, Psychiatry,
Radiology, and Sports Medicine and Surgery. Refer to "Specialties"
And "Resource Centers."

Free to use.

Medscape

www.medscape.com

Expansive clinical information covering Allergy and Immunology, Cardiology, Critical Care, Dermatology, Diabetes and Endocrinology, Family Medicine, Gastroenterology, General Surgery, Hematology-Oncology, HIV/AIDS, Infectious Diseases, Internal Medicine, Lab Medicine, Nephrology, Neurology and Neurosurgery, OB/GYN and Women's Health, Oncology, Ophthalmology, Orthopedics, Pathology and Lab Medicine, Pediatrics, Pharmacology, Primary Care, Psychiatry, Pulmonary, Radiology, Rheumatology, Surgery, Transplantation, Urology, and more. Refer to "Specialities" and "Resource Centers."

Registration required.

MDConsult

www.mdconsult.com

Expansive clinical information by Elsevier covering medical books, journals, patient education, medications, practice guidelines and more.

Subscription required.

MDLinx

www.mdlinx.com

Professional site for medical news and journal article reviews organized by subspecialty.

Registration required.

National Library of Medicine (NLM)

www.nlm.nih.gov

This is the world's largest medical library.

Free to use.

PubMed
National Library of Medicine (NLM)
www.ncbi.nlm.nih.gov/entrez/query.fcgi
Search the world's medical literature for any clinical topic.
Free to use.

Medline Plus
National Library of Medicine (NLM)
http://medlineplus.gov
Search "Health Topics" for conditions, diseases, and wellness.
Free to use.

Medical Rounds: Multimedia On-Demand
Medical Education
www.medicalrounds.com
Extensive clinical presentations covering Cardiology, Critical
Care, Endocrinology, Emergency Medicine, Infectious Diseases,
Internal Medicine, Hematology-Oncology, Nephrology, Neurology,
Pediatrics, Psychiatry, Radiology, Respirology, Rheumatology, and
Surgery.
Registration required.

COLLECTIONS BY DISEASE OR TOPIC

The New England Journal of Medicine (*NEJM*)
http://content.nejm.org/collections/
Extensive clinical materials grouped in published articles since
1996 in the *NEJM*.
Register, purchase, or subscribe.

TOPIC COLLECTIONS

British Journal of Medicine (BMJ)
http://bmj.com/cgi/collection_clinical
    Clinical and nonclinical topic article collection in the BMJ since 1998.
    Subscription or purchase required.

Journal Watch
www.jwatch.org
    Search the literature covering General, Cardiology, Dermatology, Emergency Medicine, GI, Infectious Diseases, Neurology, Pediatrics And Adolescent, Psychiatry, Women's Health, AIDS, And More.
    Subscription required.

STAT!Ref
www.statref.com
    Extensive online health care references from medical publishers and medical societies providing essential health information.
    Subscription required.

ConsultantLive
Cliggott Publishing Group
www.consultantlive.com
    Extensive clinical information but also reviews from Cancer-Network, Diagnostic Imaging, Psychiatric Time, and Applied Neurology.
    Free for healthcare professionals with registration.

National Institutes of Health (NIH)
Institutes, Centers, and Offices
www.nih.gov/icd
Comprehensive listing of all NIH institutes and centers.
Free to use.

Merck Medicus
www.merckmedicus.com/pp/us/hcp/hcp_home.jsp
Comprehensive clinical information reviewing over 7000 topics of
common medical conditions.
Registration required.

BioMed Central: The Open Access Publisher
www.biomedcentral.com
Extensive clinical topics in medicine published as journal
articles.
Free to use.

Clinical Care Options
www.clinicalcareoptions.com
Review academic resources covering HIV/AIDS, Hepatitis and
Oncology.
Registration required.

Healthlinks
University of Washington Health Sciences Libraries Seattle,
Washington
http://healthlinks.washington.edu
Comprehensive health resource
Certain sections have restricted access. User must search.

Aerospace Medicine ✍

SPACELINE
NASA Human Research and Technology
http://spaceline.usuhs.mil/current2007/index.html

Review of selected recent publications of interest in the space life sciences.

Free to use.

Aerospace Medicine Association
www.asma.org

The international leader for excellence in aerospace medicine.
Membership required.

AIDS/HIV ✍

AIDS*info*
U.S. Department of Health and Human Services
http://aidsinfo.nih.gov

Information on the treatment, prevention, and research of AIDS/HIV.
Free to use.

HIVInSite
University of California—San Francisco
http://hivinsite.ucsf.edu/

The "gateway to AIDS knowledge." It is a comprehensive site for
AIDS/HIV clinical information and research.
Free to use.

HIV/AIDS
Medscape
www.medscape.com/hiv

Comprehensive HIV/AIDS clinical topic resource.
Registration required.

HIV Pharmocology
www.hivpharmacology.com

Professional's site for information concerning HIV/AIDS pharmacology.
Free to use.

HIV Databases
http://hiv-web.lanl.gov/content/index

Academic site on HIV gene sequences, immunology, drug resistance, and vaccine trials; also contains information about the Hepatitic C Virus (HCV).

Free to use.

HIV Guide
Johns Hopkins Point-of-Care Information Technology
www.hopkins-hivguide.org

Comprehensive decision support tool for HIV/AIDS.

Free to use.

HIV/AIDS Prevention
Centers for Disease Control and Prevention (CDC)
www.cdc.gov/hiv/links.htm#resources

Comprehensive clinical resource.

Free to use.

AIDS Education Global Information Systems (AEGIS)
www.aegis.com

Extensive HIV/AIDS database.

Free to use.

HIV-Drug Interactions
The University of Liverpool—Great Britain
www.hiv-druginteractions.org

Features comprehensive pharmacology information.

Free to use.

Allergy and Immunology ✑

The Journal of Allergy and Clinical Immunology
http://journals.elsevierhealth.com/periodicals/ymai
Journal published by Elsevier for the American Academy of
Allergy, Asthma, and Immunology.
Subscription required.

The Journal of Immunology
www.jimmunol.org
Journal published by the American Association of Immunologists
for clinical and research topics.
Free to use.

Immunization
World Health Organization (WHO)
www.who.int/topics/immunization/en
Comprehensive resource on immunization.
Free to use.

Allergy and Clinical Immunology
Medscape
www.medscape.com/allergy-immunology
Comprehensive allergy and immunology clinical topic resource.
Registration required.

National Immunization Program
Centers for Disease Control and Prevention (CDC)
www.cdc.gov/vaccines/
> Extensive immunization resources for children and adults.
> Free to use.

Immunization Action Coalition
www.immunize.org
> Extensive immunization resources.
> Free to use.

Vaccine Adverse Event Reporting System (VAERS)
Centers for Disease Control and Prevention (CDC)
http://vaers.hhs.gov
> Resource for vaccine adverse events.
> Free to use.

Allergy
Medline Plus
National Library of Medicine (NLM)
www.nlm.nih.gov/medlineplus/allergy.html
> Thorough allergy link resources.
> Free to use.

Allergy and Immunology
eMedicine
**www.emedicine.com/med/ALLERGY_AND_
IMMUNOLOGY.htm**
> Excellent academic collection of clinical articles covering
> multiple topics.
> Free to use.

Immune System
National Institutes of Health (NIH)
http://health.nih.gov/search.asp?category_id=11

Immune system index on medical illnesses.

Free to use.

Alternative and Complementary Medicine ∽

National Center for Complementary and Alternative Medicine
National Institutes of Health (NIH)
http://nccam.nih.gov

    Comprehensive general information site reviewing complementary and alternative medicine research, clinical trials, health information and more.

    Free to use.

Natural Medicines Comprehensive Database
www.naturaldatabase.com

    Pharmacology database.

    Subscription required.

HerbMed
Alternative Medicine Foundation
www.herbmed.org

    Extensive herbal medicine listing.

    Free access to first 40 herbs or subscription required.

Information Resource: About Herbs, Botanicals, and Other Products
Memorial Sloan-Kettering Cancer Center— New York, New York
www.mskcc.org/mskcc/html/11570.cfm
Extensive academic integrative medicine resource.
Free to use.

Complementary/Integrative Medicine Education Resource
MD Anderson Cancer Center, Houston, Texas
www.mdanderson.org/departments/cimer
Comprehensive academic resource.
Free to use.

Alternative Medicine Review
Thorne Research, Inc.
www.thorne.com/index/mod/amr/a/amr
Academic alternative medicine journal.
Subscription required.

The Alternative Medicine Home Page
University of Pittsburgh—Pittsburgh, Pennsylvania
www.pitt.edu/~cbw/altm.html
Extensive internet link resource for alternative and complementary therapy. Must search the links.
Free to use.

Rosenthal Center for Complementary and Alternative Medicine
Columbia University—New York, New York
www.rosenthal.hs.columbia.edu/Databases.html

Extensive listing of alternative and complementary medicine databases.

Free to use, though some links may require a fee to access content.

Alternative Medicine Foundation
www.amfoundation.org

Providing responsible, evidence-based information on the integration of alternative medicine and conventional medicine.

Free to use.

Complementary and Alternative Medicine BioMed Central
www.biomedcentral.com/bmccomplementalternmed

An open-access academic journal.

Free to use.

Center for Integrative Medicine
University of Maryland, School of Medicine— Baltimore, Maryland
www.compmed.umm.edu/Databases.html

Refer to "Databases" and "CAM Resources."

Free to use.

Natural Standard
www.naturalstandard.com

An international multidisciplinary collaboration with databases covering Herb and Supplements, Interactions and much more.

Subscription required.

Drugs, Supplements, and Herbal Information
Medline Plus
National Library of Medicine (NLM)
www.nlm.nih.gov/medlineplus/druginformation.html

Search the comprehensive index.

Free to use.

Alzheimer's Disease (AD) ∽

Alzheimer's Disease (AD) and Associated Disorders
Lippincott Williams & Wilkins
www.alzheimerjournal.com
> Academic journal covering dementia disorders.
> Subscription required.

Alzheimer's Disease
Amedeo: The Medical Literature Guide
www.amedeo.com/medicine/ad.htm
> Medical literature search site.
> Free to use.

Alzheimer's Resource Room
U.S. Department of Health and Human Services
www.aoa.gov/alz/Public/alzprof/alz_prof.asp
> Good educational reference on AD.
> Free to use.

NINDS Alzheimer's Disease Information Page
National Institute of Neurological Disorders
and Stroke (NINDS)
www.ninds.nih.gov/disorders/alzheimersdisease/
alzheimersdisease.htm
> Good general reference with extensive links on AD.
> Free to use.

Alzheimer Research Forum
www.alzforum.org
> Professional site with a research focus.
> Free to use.

American Journal of Alzheimer's Disease and Other Dementias
SAGE Publications
http://aja.sagepub.com
> An academic Alzheimer's journal.
> Subscription required.

Alzheimer's Disease Education and Referral Center (ADEAR)
National Institute on Aging (NIA)
www.nia.nih.gov/Alzheimers/default.htm
> Comprehensive AD resource center.
> Free to use.

"Is It Alzheimer's Disease or Something Else?"
Postgraduate Medicine, 2005
Anna M. Barrett, MD
www.postgradmed.com/issues/2005/05_05/barrett.htm
> Good clinical differential diagnosis review.
> Free to use.

Alzheimer's Disease Resource Center
Medscape
www.medscape.com/resource/alzheimers
> Comprehensive academic resource reviewing clinical and research aspects of Alzheimer's Disease.
> Registration required.

Anemia ✑

Anemia
Medline Plus
National Library of Medicine (NLM)
www.nlm.nih.gov/medlineplus/anemia.html
> Good general anemia link resources.
> Free to use.

Anemia
Family Practice Notebook
www.fpnotebook.com/HEMCh1.htm
> Thorough primary care anemia resource.
> Free to use, but a subscription is available.

Anemia Resource Center
eMedicine
www.emedicine.com//rc/rc/pcomplete/i30/anemia.htm
> Excellent academic listing of clinical anemia articles and other resources.
> Free to use.

Sickle Cell Anemia
Medline Plus
National Library of Medicine (NLM)
www.nlm.nih.gov/medlineplus/sicklecellanemia.html
> Good general sickle cell anemia resource.
> Free to use.

The Sickle Cell Information Center
The Georgia Comprehensive Sickle Cell Center at Grady Health System—Atlanta, Georgia
www.scinfo.org
> Comprehensive resources on sickle cell anemia.
> Free to use.

Sickle Cell Disease
GeneReviews
www.geneclinics.org/query?dz=sickle
> Genetic review of sickle cell anemia.
> Free to use.

Thalassemia
Medline Plus
National Library of Medicine (NLM)
www.nlm.nih.gov/medlineplus/thalassemia.html
> Good general thalassemia review and resource.
> Free to use.

Information Center for Sickle Cell and Thalassemia Disorders
Harvard University—Boston, Massachusetts
Kenneth R. Bridges, MD
http://sickle.bwh.harvard.edu

Good clinical resource for sickle cell and thalassemia disorders.

Free to use.

Blood Diseases and Resources Information
National Heart, Lung, and Blood Institute (NHLBI)
National Institutes of Health (NIH)
www.nhlbi.nih.gov/health/public/blood/index.htm

Review general fact sheets on Anemia, Aplastic Anemia, Iron-Deficiency Anemia, Pernicious Anemia, Sickle Cell Anemia, and Thalassemia.

Free to use.

Anemia of Chronic Kidney Disease
Medscape
www.medscape.com/resource/anemia

Thorough clinical resource on anemia with kidney/renal failure. Registration required.

Hemolytic Anemia
American Family Physician, 2004
www.aafp.org/afp/20040601/2599.html

Thorough clinical review of hemolytic anemia.
Free to use.

Normocytic Anemia/Anemia of Chronic Disease
American Family Physician, 2000
www.aafp.org/afp/20001115/2255.html
> Thorough clinical review of anemia of chronic disease.
> Free to use.

Anemia of Chronic Disease
The New England Journal of Medicine (NEJM), 2005
http://content.nejm.org/cgi/content/short/352/10/1011
> Thorough clinical review of anemia of chronic disease.
> Register for free articles; purchase the article or buy a subscription for unlimited access.

National Anemia Action Council
www.anemia.org
> Comprehensive resource on anemia for patients and professionals.
> Free to use.

Cancer and Treatment-Related Anemia
National Comprehensive Cancer Network
www.nccn.org/professionals/physician_gls/PDF/anemia.pdf
> Extensive clinical review of anemia in cancer treatment.
> Usage is free, but user must download a file.

Anesthesia/Anesthesiology ⁓

GAS*net*
Global Anesthesiology Server Network
http://147.163.1.68/anestit/HomePage.html
> Academic site with clinical content for anesthesia professionals.
> Registration required.

Anesthesiology
Lippincott Williams & Wilkins
www.anesthesiology.org
> Official journal of the American Society of Anesthesiologists, Inc.
> Subscription required.

Virtual Anaesthesia Textbook
Royal Prince Alfred Hospital—Australia
www.virtual-anaesthesia-textbook.com
> Comprehensive Internet resource for anesthesia. User must search
> the links.
> Free to use.

Attention Deficit Disorder/Attention Deficit Hyperactivity Disorder (ADD/ADHD)

ADHD
National Institute of Mental Health (NIMH)
www.nimh.nih.gov/publicat/adhd.cfm
Educational review with sections covering Symptoms, Inattention, Diagnosis, Treatment and more.
Free to use.

ADHD
Medline Plus
National Library of Medicine (NLM)
www.nlm.nih.gov/medlineplus/attentiondeficit
hyperactivitydisorder.html
Comprehensive educational information with links to leading ADHD websites.
Free to use.

Attention Deficit Disorder Association
www.add.org
The world's leading adult ADHD organization. Good patient and professional resources.
Registration required.

Attention Deficit Hyperactivity Disorder (ADHD)
Centers for Disease Control and Prevention (CDC)
www.cdc.gov/ncbddd/adhd

ADHD resource with links to clinical information, treatment, research and the National Resource Center on AD/HD.

Free to use.

Attention Deficit Disorder Resources
www.addresources.org/

Extensive resources, but the user must search.

Free to use.

The ADHD e-Book
Martin L. Kutscher, MD
New York Medical College—Vahalla, New York
www.pediatricneurology.com/adhd.htm

Clinical overview on ADD/ADHD.

Free to use.

Attention Deficit Hyperactivity Disorder (ADHD)
eMedicine
www.emedicine.com/med/topic3103.htm

Academic review of ADHD.

Free to use.

Autism ✌

Autism
Medline Plus
National Library of Medicine (NLM)
www.nlm.nih.gov/medlineplus/autism.html
> Good educational autism references and resources.
> Free to use.

Autism Fact Sheet
National Institute of Neurological Disorders
and Stroke (NINDS)
National Institutes of Health (NIH)
www.ninds.nih.gov/disorders/autism/detail_autism.htm
> Thorough general autism review.
> Free to use.

Autism Spectrum Disorders
Medscape
www.medscape.com/resource/autism
> Excellent academic collection of autism resources.
> Registration required.

Pervasive Developmental Disorder: Autism
eMedicine
www.emedicine.com/ped/topic180.htm

Academic review of autism and related disorders. Review "Autism Resource Center."

Free to use.

Autism
Online Mendelian Inheritance in Man (OMIM)
National Center for Biotechnology Information (NCBI)
www.ncbi.nlm.nih.gov/entrez/dispomim.cgi?id=209850

Comprehensive genetic review on autism.

Free to use.

Autism
National Center on Birth Defects and
Developmental Disabilities
Centers for Disease Control and Prevention (CDC)
www.cdc.gov/ncbddd/autism/actearly

Excellent review for important developmental milestones for children and possible developmental problems.

Free to use.

Autism Information Center
Centers for Disease Control and Prevention (CDC)
www.cdc.gov/ncbddd/autism/index.htm

Good resource selection on autism.

Free to use.

Knowledge Path: Autism Spectrum Disorders
Maternal and Child Health Library
Georgetown University—Washington, DC
www.mchlibrary.info/KnowledgePaths/kp_autism.html

Excellent educational collection of autism resources, but user must search links.

Free to use.

Autism Spectrum Disorders
National Institute of Mental Health (NIMH)
National Institutes of Health (NIH)
www.nimh.nih.gov/publicat/autism.cfm

Detailed autism review.

Free to use.

Journal of Autism and Developmental Disorders
SpringerLink
www.springerlink.com/content/1573-3432

Academic journal reviewing clinical and research information on developmental disorders.

Subscription required.

"Autism: The Hidden Epidemic"
MSNBC
www.msnbc.msn.com/id/6844737

News report covering autism and related clinical issues.

Free to use.

Autism
Neurosciences for Kids
University of Washington—Seattle, Washington
http://faculty.washington.edu/chudler/aut.html

Excellent educational resource site.

Free to use.

Autism
American Academy of Pediatrics
www.aap.org/healthtopics/autism.cfm

Excellent professional resource on autism.

Free to use.

Bioethics/Medical Ethics ❧

Kennedy Institute of Ethics
Georgetown University—Washington, DC
http://bioethics.georgetown.edu
> Extensive library and information services for bioethics research.
> Free to use.

Bioethics Resources on the Web
National Institutes of Health (NIH)
http://bioethics.od.nih.gov
> Extensive information database.
> Free to use.

Ethics Updates
University of San Diego—San Diego, CA
http://ethics.sandiego.edu
> Comprehensive site covering areas of Ethical Theory, Resources, and Applied Ethics.
> Free to use.

Journal of Medical Ethics
BMJ Publishing Group Ltd.
http://jme.bmj.com
> Leading medical ethics journal.
> Subscription required.

BMC Medical Ethics
BioMed Central
www.biomedcentral.com/bmcmedethics
> Open access journal to medical ethics topics.
> Free to use.

Advance Medical Directives
University of Arkansas for Medical Sciences
Little Rock, Arkansas
www.uams.edu/patienteducation/Handouts/
advance_medical_directives.pdf
> Medical decision making information for patients.
> May vary by state law.
> Free to use, but user must search the links.

Advance Directives
Medline Plus
National Library of Medicine (NLM)
www.nlm.nih.gov/medlineplus/advancedirectives.html
> Good educational resource.
> Free to use, but user must search the links.

Advances Directives
The Patient Education Forum
The American Geriatric Society
www.americangeriatrics.org/education/Forum/
advance.shtml
> Good resource with links to each state's requirements.
> Free to use.

Bioterrorism/Nuclear, Biological, and Chemical ✍

Emergency Preparedness and Response
Centers for Disease Control and Prevention (CDC)
www.bt.cdc.gov/bioterrorism
> Excellent site on agents, diseases, and other threats.
> Free to use.

Bioterrorism
World Health Organization (WHO)
www.who.int/topics/bioterrorism/en
> Excellent review. Search for agents under "HealthTopics."
> Free to use.

Biological Warfare and Its Cutaneous Manifestations
The Electronic Textbook of Dermatology
The Internet Dermatology Society, Inc.
Thomas W. McGovern, MD, MAJ, MC
George W. Christopher, LTC, USAF, MC
http://telemedicine.org/biowar/biologic.htm
> Great images of bioterrorism skin diseases.
> Free to use.

CBRNE-Biological Warfare Agents
eMedicine
www.emedicine.com/emerg/topic853.htm
> Excellent academic review.
> Free to use.

Biodefense and Bioterrorism Medline Plus
National Institutes of Health (NIH)
**www.nlm.nih.gov/medlineplus/biodefenceand-
bioterrorism.html**
> Thorough resource covering bioterrorism.
> Free to use, but user must search links.

NIAID Biodefense Research
National Institute of Allergy and Infectious Diseases (NIAID)
www3.niaid.nih.gov/biodefense
> Biodefense information for biomedical researchers, the public, and the media.
> Free to use.

Bioterrorism
Medscape
www.medscape.com/resource/bioterr
> Thorough clinical resource on bioterrorism.
> Registration required.

Public Health Image Library (PHIL)
Centers for Disease Control and Prevention (CDC)
http://phil.cdc.gov/phil/home.asp
> Excellent academic resource. Review "PHIL Collections."
> Free to use.

JEFFSelects: Bioterrorism
Thomas Jefferson University—Philadelphia, Pennsylvania
http://jeffline.jefferson.edu/SML/JEFFSelects/anthrax.html

Excellent link list of educational resources for bioterrorism.

Some materials are free, but others require subscription or code access.

NBC-Links
www.nbc-links.com

Extensive resources for nuclear, biological, and chemical materials.

Free to use.

Chemical Warfare Agents
www.opcw.org/resp/html/cwagents.html

Detailed review of nerve agents, mustard agents, hydrogen cyanide, arsines, psychotomimetic agents, toxins, and more.

Free to use.

Center for Biologic Counterterrorism and Emerging Diseases
MedStar Health Group
www.bepast.org

Extensive bioterrorism and other infectious disease resources.

Free to use.

Birth Defects ❦

Developmental and Genetic Diseases
Geneva Foundation for Medical Education and Research
www.gfmer.ch/genetic_diseases_v2/index.php
  Extensive listing with photos of developmental and genetic diseases.
  Free to use.

Genetics/Birth Defects
Medline Plus
National Library of Medicine (NLM)
www.nlm.nih.gov/medlineplus/geneticsbirthdefects.html
  Excellent general resource.
  Free to use.

Birth Defects
Centers for Disease Control and Prevention (CDC)
www.cdc.gov/node.do/id/0900f3ec8000dffe
  Good clinical resource.
  Free to use.

International Clearinghouse for Birth Defects
www.icbdsr.org
  International organization for birth defects surveillance and research. Review "Web Guide," and "Resources."
  Free to use.

National Center on Birth Defects and Developmental Disabilities (NCBDDD)
Centers for Disease Control and Prevention (CDC)
www.cdc.gov/ncbddd
>Good general resource.
>Free to use.

Birth Defects
Health on the Net Foundation (HON)
**http://debussy.hon.ch/cgi-bin/find?1+submit+
birth_defects**
>Extensive listing of birth defect sites. User must search.
>Free to use, but certain sites may require registration or a fee.

Birth Defects and Developmental Disabilities
National Institute of Child Health and Human Development (NICHD)
**www.nichd.nih.gov/womenshealth/research/pregbirth/
birthdefects.cfm**
>Detailed birth defects resource.
>Free to use.

National Birth Defects Prevention Network
www.nbdpn.org
>Excellent reference. Review under "Resources" on the website.
>Registration required for membership.

Developmental Disabilities
Medline Plus
National Library of Medicine (NLM)
www.nlm.nih.gov/medlineplus/developmental disabilities.html

Thorough listing of developmental disability resources.
Free to use.

Breast Cancer ✍

Breast Cancer Resource Center
Medscape
www.medscape.com/resource/breastcancer
Academic resource for breast cancer.
Registration required.

Breast Cancer
Medline Plus
National Library of Medicine (NLM)
www.nlm.nih.gov/medlineplus/breastcancer.html
Good general resource.
Free to use.

Breast Cancer
National Cancer Institute (NCI)
National Institutes of Health (NIH)
http://wwwicic.nci.nih.gov/cancertopics/types/breast
Extensive breast cancer resources.
Free to use.

BRCA1 and BRCA2 Heredity Breast/Ovarian Cancer
Gene Reviews
www.genetests.org/query?dz=brca1
Academic review on genetic mutations.
Free to use.

Breast Cancer
Online Mendelian Inheritance in Man (OMIM)
www.ncbi.nlm.nih.gov/entrez/dispomim.cgi?id=114480
Detailed review of the genetics on breast cancer.
Free to use.

Breast Cancer Collection
The New England Journal of Medicine (NEJM)
http://content.nejm.org/cgi/collection/breast_cancer
Academic journal articles on the topic of breast cancer.
Register, purchase, or subscribe required.

Assessing Breast Cancer Risk
Postgraduate Medicine Online, 2004
Larissa A. Korde, MD, MPH et al
www.postgradmed.com/issues/2004/10_04/
korde.htm
Symposium on breast cancer that includes "Managing Early
Breast Cancer" and "Care of the Breast Cancer Survivor."
Free to use.

Breast Cancer (Nonmetastatic/Metastatic)
British Medical Journal
Clinical Evidence
www.clinicalevidence.com/ceweb/index.jsp
Breast-cancer literature review that is evidence-based medicine.
Click "Condition," then "Oncology" and "Breast Cancer."
Register, purchase, or subscribe.

Breast Cancer
Centers for Disease Control and Prevention (CDC)
www.cdc.gov/cancer/breast/links.htm

Extensive breast cancer links. User must search the site for information.

Often free to use, but certain links may require registration or a fee.

Breast Cancer
National Cancer Institute (NCI)
National Institutes of Health (NIH)
www.cancer.gov/cancertopics/wyntk/breast

Expansive breast cancer resource covering all disease aspects.
Free to use.

OncoLink
Abramson Cancer Center
University of Pennsylvania—Philadelphia, Pennsylvania
http://oncolink.upenn.edu/types

Click "Breast Cancer" for a thorough discussion.
Free to use.

Breast Cancer Online
www.bco.org

Educational service for medical professionals reviewing breast cancer.
Registration required.

Breast Cancer
New York Online Access to Health (NOAH)
www.noah-health.org/en/cancer/types/breast

A good general resource for patients.
Often free to use, but certain links may require registration or fee.

Breast Cancer Risk Assessment Tool
National Cancer Institute (NCI)
www.cancer.gov/bcrisktool

An interactive tool for measuring the risk of invasive breast cancer.

Free to use.

Breast Cancer—Male
eMedicine
www.emedicine.com/RADIO/topic115.htm

Academic review and other resources for researching male breast cancer.

Free to use.

Cardiology/Heart Disease ∾

Cardiosource
American College of Cardiology (ACC)
www.cardiosource.com

Comprehensive academic site covering cardiology. See "Clinical Collections," "Guidelines and Trials," and more.

Some materials are free, but a fee may be required for others.

Cardiology
Medscape
www.medscape.com/cardiology

Online cardiology resources.

Registration required.

Cardiology
eMedicine
www.emedicine.com/med/CARDIOLOGY.htm

Extensive academic resources covering multiple topics.

Free to use.

Cardiology
Journal Watch
http://cardiology.jwatch.org

Review selected cardiology journals.

Subscription or purchase required.

Cardiology Clinical Statements/Guidelines
American College of Cardiology (ACC)
www.acc.org/qualityandscience/clinical/statements.htm
   Comprehensive collection of clinical cardiology guidelines.
   Free to use.

National Heart, Lung, and Blood Institute (NHLBI)
National Institutes of Health (NIH)
www.nhlbi.nih.gov
   Extensive clinical cardiology resources.
   Free to use.

Cardiology Library
Medscape
www.medscape.com/cardiology/journals
   Extensive cardiac resources.
   Fee required for access to most journals.

Cardiovascular Disorders
BioMed Central
www.biomedcentral.com/bmccardiovascdisord/
   Online cardiovascular journal.
   Free to use.

Cardiology Rounds
Cardiology Division at Brigham and Women's Hospital—
Boston, Massachusetts
www.cardiologyrounds.org
   Excellent cardiovascular clinical resource reviewing different
patient heart diseases.
   Free to use.

Cardiovascular Diseases
The New England Journal of Medicine (NEJM)
http://content.nejm.org/cgi/collection/
cardiovascular_diseases

>Extensive cardiovascular collection by disease or topic.
>Registration, purchase, or subscription required.

Current Opinion in Cardiology
Lippincott Williams & Wilkins
www.co-cardiology.com

>Keep current with cardiology journal publications.
>Subscription or purchase required.

Journal of American College of Cardiology
http://content.onlinejacc.org

>Professional academic journal published by the American College
>of Cardiology.
>Subscription required.

Cardiology
MyMedline.com
www.atlife.com/medline/cardiology.php3

>Search cardiology journals.
>Often free to use, but some journals require fees.

Chest Pain Perspectives
Dade Behring
www.chestpainperspectives.com

>Extensive educational resource. Review "Medical Professional"
>section.
>Registration required.

CVspectrum.org
www.cvspectrum.org
>A comprehensive dyslipidemic and atherosclerosis resource.
>Registration required.

Liped Resource Center
eMedicine
www.emedicine.com/rc/rc/pfeatured/i1/lipid.htm
>An educational resource on global cardiac risk reduction.
>Free to use.

Lipids Online
Baylor College of Medicine—Houston, Texas
http://lipidsonline.org
>"Educational Resources in Atherosclerosis" utilizes a slide
library and Continuing Medical Information Education.
>Free to use.

Congential Heart Disease
Yale University School of Medicine—
New Haven, Connecticut
http://info.med.yale.edu/intmed/cardio/chd
>Extensive collection of CHD conditions.
>Free to use.

"Cardiology: Congenital Heart Diseases, Their Study and Treatment" Oliver W. Caminos, MD
www.redtail.net/owc
>Comprehensive review of CHD conditions with detailed drawings
of individual disorders.
>Free to use.

Cardiac Rhythm Management
Medscape
www.medscape.com/resource/crm
Cardiac arrhythmia resources.
Registration required.

Arrhythmia
American Heart Association (AHA)
www.americanheart.org/presenter.jhtml?identifier=82
Comprehensive arrhythmias information.
Free to use.

ArizonaCERT-Drug-Induced Arrhythmias
University of Arizona—Tucson, Arizona
www.qtdrugs.org
Excellent resource on pro-arrhythmia drugs.
Free to use.

Einthoven
Advances in Cardiac Arrhythmias
www.xagena.it/einthoven/index.html
Extensive cardiac resources on arrhythmias.
Free to use.

Implantable.com
www.implantable.com
A pacemaker and defibrillator site index.
Free to use.

EKG Rounds
MDchoice
www.mdchoice.com/ekg/ekg.asp
EKG tracings with explanations.
Free to use.

EKG World Encyclopedia
McGill University—Montreal, Canada
http://sprojects.mmi.mcgill.ca/heart/egcyhome.html
EKG educational archive file.
Free to use.

ECG Library
www.ecglibrary.com/ecghome.html
Good collection of ECG tracings with clinical explanations.
Free to use.

Women-Related Statements/Guidelines
American Heart Association (AHA)
www.americanheart.org/presenter.jhtml?
identifier=3020323
Collection of evidence-based clinical statements and guidelines
for women. Check "Go Red for Women."
Free to use.

American Society of Hypertension, Inc.
www.ash-us.org
"About Hypertension" is an excellent hypertension resource.
Free to use.

The Heart Surgery Forum
www.hsforum.com
> An online multimedia journal cardiothoracic surgery covering.
> Free to use, but *Heart Surgery Forum* journal requires subscription.

CTS*Net*
www.ctsnet.org
> The cardiothoracic surgery online network.
> Contains many free resources, but membership/purchases may be required.

VascularWeb
The Society for Vascular Surgery
www.vascularweb.org
> Good vascular clinical information for professionals and patients.
> Some materials are free but certain access requires membership.

ECHO in Context
Duke University Center for ECHO—Durham, North Carolina
www.echoincontext.com
> Comprehensive cardiac ECHO resource.
> Free to use.

Chronic Obstructive Pulmonary Disease (COPD) ∽

The Global Initiative for Chronic Obstructive Lung Disease (GOLD)
www.goldcopd.com
> Excellent resource. Review "Guidelines and Resources."
> Free to use.

Chronic Obstructive Pulmonary Disease (COPD) Medline Plus
National Library of Medicine (NLM)
www.nlm.nih.gov/medlineplus/copdchronicobstructive pulmonarydisease.html
> Thorough collection of resources.
> Free to use.

COPD and Emphysema
eMedicine
www.emedicine.com/emerg/topic99.htm
> Excellent international COPD evidence-based guidelines and more.
> Free to use.

Chronic Obstructive Pulmonary Disease (COPD)
Medscape Resource Centers
http:dev.ersnet.org
Good COPD resources.
Registration required.

European Respiratory Society
http://dev.ersnet.org
Review "Inside the ERS" with "Learning Resources" and "ERS Guidelines" for information on COPD and more.
Fee required for access to certain parts of the site.

National Lung Health Education Program
www.nlhep.org
Excellent education site with resources on tobacco control, smoking cessation, lung cancer, breathing tests and more.
Free to use.

COPD-Alert
www.copd-alert.com
Excellent COPD resource.
Free to use.

COPD Guidelines
American Thoracic Society (ATS)
www.thoracic.org/sections/copd/index.html
Lists the standards for the diagnosis and management of patients with COPD.
Also review "Clinical Information."
Fees required for access to certain parts of the site.

Chronic Obstructive Pulmonary Disease (COPD)
Fact Sheet
American Lung Association (ALA)
www.lungusa.org/site/pp.asp?c=dvLUK9OOE&b=35020
Extensive fact sheet on COPD.

Free to use.

Chronic Obstructive Pulmonary Disease (COPD)
Centers for Disease Control and Prevention (CDC)
www.cdc.gov/nceh/airpollution/copd/copdfaq.htm
Fact sheet covering COPD and related resources.

Free to use.

Chronic Obstructive Airways Disease
Thorax Online
http://thorax.bmj.com/cgi/collection/chronic_
obstructive_airways
Extensive collection of articles on COPD and related topics.

Fee required.

Pulmonary Rehabilitation
eMedicine
www.emedicine.com/pmr/topic181.htm
Excellent clinical review covering the components of pulmonary
rehabilitation.

Free to use.

Portable Oxygen: A User's Perspective
www.portableoxygen.org
Good reference site on oxygen usage, devices for delivery, and more.

Free to use.

International Ventilator Users Network (IVUN)

www.ventusers.org

Indepth information covering all the aspects for home mechanical ventilation.

Free to use, but fees may be required for certain content.

Chronic Obstructive Pulmonary Disease Symposium Postgraduate Medicine, 2005

www.postgradmed.com/issues/2005/03_05/ comm_petty.htm

Academic review of COPD with opening commentary by renowned pulmonary physician Thomas L. Petty, MD.

Free to use.

Clinical Calculators ✎

Clinical Calculators and Scoring Systems
MDchoice
www.mdchoice.com/calculators.asp

Online Clinical Calculator
Bayesian Analysis Model
Medical College of Wisconsin
www.intmed.mcw.edu/clincalc/bayes.html

Charlie's Clinical Calculator
www.medcalc.com

The Clinician's Ultimate Reference
Clinical Calculators
www.globalrph.com/calculators.htm

Online Clinical Calculators
MedStudents
Richard Z. Toptani, MD
www.medstudents.com.br/calculat/index2.htm

Medal: The Medical Algorithms Project
Institute for Algorithmic Medicine—Houston, Texas
www.medal.org
> Extensive resource.
> Registration required.

MedCalc3000
http://medcalc3000.com
> Extensive resource with online, pocket PC, stand-alone, and BlackBerry versions.
> Purchase required.

Acid-Base Calculator
MedCalc
www.medcalc.com/acidbase.html

Clinical Trials ✌

Using these sites, search for private or federal clinical trials.
Free to use.

ClinicalTrials.gov
National Institutes of Health (NIH)
www.clinicaltrials.gov

ClinicalTrials.com
www.clinicaltrials.com

CenterWatch
Clinical Trials Listing Service
www.centerwatch.com

Cancer Trials Support Unit (CTSU)
National Cancer Institute (NCI)
www.ctsu.org

Clinical Trials
National Cancer Institute (NCI)
www.cancer.gov/clinicaltrials

International Maternal Pediatric Adolescent AIDS
Clinical Trials Group (IMPAACT)
http://pactg.s-3.com/impaact.htm

Colorectal Cancer ∽

Colorectal Cancer
Medscape
www.medscape.com/resource/colcancer
Excellent clinical resource.
· Registration required.

Colon Cancer, Adenocarcinoma
eMedicine
www.emedicine.com/MED/topic413.htm
Thorough clinical review of colon cancer and related topics.
Free to use.

Colon and Rectal Cancer
National Cancer Institute (NCI)
National Institutes of Health (NIH)
www.cancer.gov/cancertopics/types/colon-and-rectal
Excellent review of colorectal cancer.
Free to use.

Colorectal Cancer
Medline Plus
National Library of Medicine (NLM)
www.nlm.nih.gov/medlineplus/colorectalcancer.html
Excellent resources for colorectal cancer.
Free to use.

Images from the Colon and Ileum
EndoAtlas
www.endoatlas.com/atlas_co.html

Excellent images. Review "Malignant Tumors."

Free to use.

Colorectal Cancer
OncoLink
University of Pennsylvania—Philadelphia, Pennsylvania
http://oncolink.upenn.edu

Excellent clinical review of colorectal cancer. Go to "Types of Cancer," and then click "C" for colorectal cancer.

Free to use.

Congestive Heart Failure (CHF) ∾

Heart Failure
Medscape
www.medscape.com/resource/heartfailure
Extensive resource on heart failure and related topics.
Registration required.

Congestive Heart Failure and Pulmonary Edema
eMedicine
www.emedicine.com/emerg/topic108.htm
Thorough clinical review on CHF and related clinical topics.
Free to use.

Heart Failure
eMedicine
www.emedicine.com/med/topic3552.htm
Thorough clinical review of heart failure. Review "Heart Failure Resource Center."
Free to use.

Heart Failure
Medline Plus
National Library of Medicine (NLM)
www.nlm.nih.gov/medlineplus/heartfailure.html
Good resource for CHF.
Free to use.

Chronic Heart Failure in Adults
ACC/AHA Practice Guidelines, 2005 Update
The American College of Cardiology
http://content.onlinejacc.org/cgi/content/full/46/6/1116

Summary article on practice guidelines for chronic heart failure.
Free to use.

Heart Failure
New England Journal of Medicine (NEJM)
http://content.nejm.org/cgi/collection/heart_failure

Collection of academic articles on CHF.
Subscription or purchase required for article access.

Heart Failure
The Merck Manual
www.merck.com/mmpe/sec07/ch074/ch074b.html

Thorough review of heart failure and cardiomyopathies.
Free to use.

Critical Care/Intensive Care Medicine ∽

Critical Care
http://ccforum.com
Academic site with Dr. Jean-Louis Vincent as Editor-in-Chief, for Subscription required.

PedsCCM: The Pediatric Critical Care Website
http://pedsccm.org
Spectacular educational site—review "Clinical Resources" and so much more.
Free to use, but some material may require purchase.

Virtual Pediatric Intensive Care Unit
www.picu.net
Extensive academic information.
Free to use.

Society of Critical Care Medicine
www.sccm.org
Professional society for critical care medicine. Review "Professional Development," "Public Health and Policy," and so much more.
Some materials are free, but membership in this professional organization is required.

Critical Care Medicine
Lippincott Williams & Wilkins
www.ccmjournal.com
> Official journal of the Society of Critical Care Medicine.
> Subscription required.

Intensive Care Medicine
SpringerLink
www.springerlink.com/content/100428
> Academic journal reviewing all aspects of critical care
medicine.
> Subscription required.

ICU Delirium and Cognitive Impairment Study Group
Vanderbilt University Medical Center—
Nashville, Tennessee
www.icudelirium.org/delirium
> Extensive ICU delirium resources.
> Free to use.

NHLBI ARDS Network
www.ardsnet.org
> Extensive Acute Respiratory Distress Syndrome (ARDS)
resource.
> Free to use.

IntensiveCare.com
www.intensivecare.com
> Resources for supporting evidence-based medicine in critical
care.
> Free to use.

Advances in Sepsis
www.advancesinsepsis.com
Commentary and analysis on advances in the understanding and treatment of sepsis.
Free to use.

Sepsis: Pathophysiology and Treatment
Medscape
www.medscape.com/resource/sepsis
Clinical review of sepsis.
Registration required.

Critical Care Medicine
American Thoracic Society (ATS)
**www.thoracic.org/sections/clinical-information/
critical-care/index.html**
Excellent clinical resources.
Free to use, but fee required for membership to the society.

International Collaboration for Excellence in
Critical Care Medicine (ICE-CCM)
http://ice-ccm.medtau.org
"Collaborative effort to enhance excellence in crtical care medicine. . . ." Review "CCM Resources," "Links," and more.
Free to use.

Pediatric Critical Care
Medical Calculators
Cornell University—New York, New York
**www-users.med.cornell.edu/~spon/picu/calc/
index.htm**

Pediatric CCM clinical tools.

Free to use.

Pediatric Critical Care
eMedicine
www.emedicine.com/ped/CRITICAL_CARE.htm

Academic collection of pediatric crtitical care articles.

Free to use.

Institute for Healthcare Improvement Critical Care
www.ihi.org/IHI/topics/criticalcare

A comprehensive resource for implementing improvements in critical care.

Registration required.

Adult Critical Care
eMedicine
www.emedicine.com/med/CRITICAL_CARE.htm

Academic collection of adult critical care articles.

Free to use.

Cross-Cultural Health/
Minority Health ✧

The Office of Minority Health (OMH)
U.S. Department of Health and Human Services
www.omhrc.gov

To improve and protect the health of racial and ethnic minority populations.

Free to use.

Unequal Treatment: Confronting Racial and Ethnic Disparities in Health Care (2003)
The National Academies Press
http://books.nap.edu/catalog.php?record_id=10260

Extensive review of health care disparities with racial and ethnic minorities.

Free online, or purchase a hard copy of the text or CD-ROM.

EthnoMed
University of Washington—Seattle, Washington
http://ethnomed.org

Excellent resource for information about health care of immigrants to Seattle, Washington and the United States.

Free to use.

Cultural Competence Resources for Health Care Providers
Health Resources and Services Administration
U.S. Department of Health and Human Services
www.hrsa.gov/culturalcompetence

Excellent resource.

Free to use.

Factline
National Library of Medicine (NLM)/
Meharry Medical College
www.meharry.org/FL

Excellent presentation of information regarding health disparities faced by women, minority groups, the elderly, and more.

Free to use.

Think Cultural Health
U.S. Department of Health and Human Services
www.thinkculturalhealth.org

CME programs and resources on culture competency health care.

Free to use.

National Center for Cultural Competence
Georgetown University—Washington, DC
www11.georgetown.edu/research/gucchd/nccc/
index.html

Excellent resource.

Free to use.

Office of Minority Health
Centers for Disease Control and Prevention (CDC)
www.cdc.gov/omhd
> Great reference site.
> Free to use.

Multicultural Health
Queensland Government—Australia
www.health.qld.gov.au/multicultural
> Excellent cross-cultural health site. Users must search the links.
> Free to use.

The Provider's Guide of Quality and Culture
http://erc.msh.org
> Electronic resource for cross-cultural care. Go to "Quick Links,"
> and select the title.
> Registration required.

Medscape
Health Diversity
www.medscape.com/resource/healthdiverse
> Thorough review on health diversity and its delivery.
> Registration required.

Dermatology/Skin Disease ✐

Dermatology Databases
University of Iowa—Iowa City, Iowa
http://tray.dermatology.uiowa.edu/DermDB.htm

Comprehensive academic link site for dermatology. User must search links.

Free to use but fee required for certain access.

Dermatology Image Atlas
Johns Hopkins University—Baltimore, Maryland
www.dermatlas.com/derm

Over 8,000 images and more. Review "DermAtlas Links."

Free to use.

Dermatology Online Journal
http://dermatology.cdlib.org

Open-access dermatology journal.

Free to use.

Dermatology
eMedicine
www.emedicine.com/derm

Extensive academic resource on skin diseases.

Free to use.

Journal of the American Academy of Dermatology
Elsevier
www.eblue.org
> Professional dermatology journal.
> Subscription required.

DermNet
www.dermnet.com
> Excellent database for skin diseases.
> Free to use.

Diabetes Mellitus ∾

Diabetes Mellitus, Type 1(DM1)—A Review
eMedicine
www.emedicine.com/emerg/topic133.htm
> Excellent academic review.
> Free to use.

Diabetes Mellitus, Type 2(DM2)—A Review
eMedicine
www.emedicine.com/emerg/topic134.htm
> Excellent academic review.
> Free to use.

Diabetic Ketoacidosis
eMedicine
www.emedicine.com/emerg/topic135.htm
> Excellent academic review.
> Free to use.

"Gestational Diabetes Mellitus"
The New England Journal of Medicine (*NEJM*), 1999
Siri L. Kjos, M.D. and Thomas A. Buchanan, M.D.
**http://content.nejm.org/cgi/content/extract/
341/23/1749**
> Excellent clinical review.
> Registration, purchase, or subscription required.

Diabetes Type I
Medline Plus
National Library of Medicine (NLM)
www.nlm.nih.gov/medlineplus/diabetestype1.html
> Good general resource.
> Free to use.

Diabetes
Medline Plus
National Library of Medicine (NLM)
www.nlm.nih.gov/medlineplus/diabetes.html
> Good general resource.
> Free to use.

Introduction to Diabetes
National Diabetes Information Clearinghouse (NDIC)
National Institute of Diabetes and Digestive and
Kidney Diseases (NIDDK)
http://diabetes.niddk.nih.gov/intro/index.htm
> General review of DM1, DM2, Children and Pregnancy.
> Free to use.

Diabetes Mellitus Complications
Family Practice Notebook
www.fpnotebook.com/END16.htm
> Extensive general practice review of diabetes complications.
> Free to use, but a subscription option is available.

Diabetic Microvascular Complications
Medscape
www.medscape.com/resource/microvascular
   Review of diabetic microvascular complications and interventions for its control.
   Registration required.

Diabetes Neuropathies and Neuromuscular Disorders
Washington University—St. Louis, Missouri
www.neuro.wustl.edu/neuromuscular/nother/diabetes.htm
   Comprehensive outline overview.
   Free to use.

Diabetes Mellitus, Insulin-Dependent (IDDM)
Online Mendelian Inheritance in Man (OMIM)
www.ncbi.nlm.nih.gov/entrez/dispomim.cgi?id=222100
   Excellent genetic review of diabetes mellitus.
   Free to use.

Skin Problems Associated with Diabetes Mellitus
DermNet NZ
http://dermnetnz.org/systemic/diabetes.html#dd
   Clinical overview of skin disorders with diabetes mellitus.
   Free to use.

Diabetes Mellitus and Pregnancy
Access Medicine
McGraw-Hill
www.accessmedicine.com/content.aspx?aid=2385290
   Excellent clinical review.
   Subscription required.

Joslin's Diabetes Mellitus, 2004
Lippincott Williams & Wilkins
www.lww.com/product/?978-0-7817-2796-9

The "bible" of diabetes mellitus.

Purchase required.

International Textbook of Diabetes Mellitus, 2004
R. A. DeFronzo, et al
John Wiley & Sons, Inc.
**www.wiley.com/WileyCDA/WileyTitle/
productCd-0471486558.html**

Comprehensive reference on diabetes mellitus.

Purchase required.

National Diabetes Education Program
National Institutes of Health (NIH)
www.ndep.nih.gov

Very useful information for diabetic patients and health care professionals.

Free to use.

Eldercare ❧

Elder Abuse
Medline Plus
National Library of Medicine (NLM)
www.nlm.nih.gov/medlineplus/elderabuse.html
    Excellent selection of resources on elder abuse.
    Free to use.

Eldercare Locator
U.S. Department of Health and Human Services
www.eldercare.gov
    Extensive information on senior services.
    Free to use.

Senior Citizens' Resources
USA.gov
www.usa.gov/Topics/Seniors.shtml
    Extensive resources for seniors.
    Free to use.

Administration on Aging
U.S. Department of Health and Human Services
www.aoa.dhhs.gov
    Comprehensive federal website on resources for older Americans.
    Free to use.

The Eldercare Team
www.eldercareteam.com
> Good site for eldercare caregivers on questions and answers, resources, and support.
> Free to use.

BenefitsCheckUp
The National Council on Aging
www.benefitscheckup.org
> Resources devoted to helping seniors find benefit programs.
> Free to use.

Gilbert Guide
www.gilbertguide.com
> Reliable resource of detailed information on senior care facilities and resources.
> Free to use.

Health Assistance Partnership
www.hapnetwork.org
> Comprehensive resources to assist Medicare beneficiaries with health care.
> Free to use.

Emergency Medicine ∽

National Center for Emergency Medicine Informatics (NCEMI)
http://ncemi.org

ED (Emergency Department) information site. Many useful clinical resources.

Free to use, but site in development.

Emergency Medicine
eMedicine
www.emedicine.com/emerg

Excellent and extensive resource.

Free to use.

The Pediatric Emergency Medicine Database
http://researchinpem.homestead.com

Online pediatric emergency database.

Free to use.

Emergency Preparedness and Response
Centers for Disease Control and Prevention (CDC)
www.bt.cdc.gov

Excellent site for bioterrorism agents, diseases, and other threats.

Free to use.

Natural Hazards Center
University of Colorado, Boulder, Colorado
www.colorado.edu/hazards/library
HAZLIT database and search engine.
Free to use.

Pandemic Flu
U.S. Department of Health and Human Services
www.pandemicflu.gov
Comprehensive resource on seasonal flu, avian flu, and pandemic flu.
Free to use.

Epidemic and Pandemic Alert and Response (EPR)
World Health Organization (WHO)
www.who.int/csr/disease/avian_influenza/en
Comprehensive avian influenza resource.
Free to use.

Disaster! Finder
National Aeronautics and Space Administration (NASA)
http://disasterfinder.gsfc.nasa.gov
Comprehensive resource for disaster links.
Free to use.

Earth Observatory
Natural Hazards
NASA
http://earthobservatory.nasa.gov/NaturalHazards
Excellent collection of satellite photos from worldwide natural
hazards plus disaster links.
Free to use.

Endocrinology/Hormone Disorders ✍

Endotext.org
www.endotext.org
Academic endocrine website.
Free to use.

Cardiovascular Diabetology
BioMed Central
www.cardiab.com
Covers all aspects of diabetes and cardiovascular disease in an online journal.
Free to use.

Endocrinology
The Endocrinology Society
http://endo.endojournals.org
Academic endocrine journal.
Subscription required.

Endocrinology
eMedicine
www.emedicine.com/med/ENDOCRINOLOGY.htm
Excellent academic resource.
Free to use.

The Journal of Clinical Endocrinology and Metabolism
The Endocrine Society
http://jcem.endojournals.org
>Academic endocrine journal.
>Subscription required.

Endocrinology Notebook
Family Practice Notebook
www.fpnotebook.com/END.htm
>Primary care endocrine review.
>Free to use, but a subscription option is available.

Current Opinion in Endocrinology, Diabetes, and Obesity
Lippincott Williams & Wilkins
www.co-endocrinology.com
>Academic endocrine journal.
>Subscription required.

Diabetes and Endocrinology
Medscape
www.medscape.com/diabetes-endocrinology
>Good clinical resource.
>Registration required.

Endocrinology
Pediatrics
http://pediatrics.aappublications.org/cgi/collection/endocrinology
>Academic endocrine journal review.
>Subscription required.

End-of-Life Care/
Palliative Care ∽

End of Life/Palliative Education
Resource Center (EPERC)
The Medical College of Wisconsin—
Milwaukee, Wisconsin
www.eperc.mcw.edu
> Extensive academic information.
> Free to use.

The Center to Advance Palliative Care
The Robert Wood Johnson Foundation
www.capc.org
> All the essentials for palliative care.
> Registration and/or purchase for materials.

When Children Die: Improving Palliative
and End-of-Life Care for Children
and Their Families
The National Academies Press
Marilyn J. Field and Richard E. Behrman, 2003
www.nap.edu/catalog.php?record_id=10390
> An essential informative book for everyone involved in pediatric
> palliative care/end-of-life care delivery.
> Purchase required.

The Initiative for Pediatric Palliative Care
www.ippcweb.org
>Extensive educational materials.
>Free to use.

Palliative Care Policy Center
www.medicaring.org
>Extensive resources on end-of-life care.
>Free to use.

Growthhouse
www.growthhouse.org
>A gateway to resources for life-threatening illness and end-of-life care.
>Free to use.

On Our Own Terms: Moyers on Dying
PBS
www.thirteen.org/onourownterms
>Educational television series on end-of-life care.
>Free to use.

End-of-Life Care Consensus Panel
American College of Physicians (ACP)
www.acponline.org/ethics/papers.htm
>Extensive professional resource.
>Free to use but certain sections may require membership or purchase.

EndLink
Robert H. Lurie Comprehensive Cancer Center
Northwestern University—Chicago, Illinois
http://endlink.lurie.northwestern.edu

An excellent educational resource for people involved in end-of-life care.

Free to use.

Journal of Palliative Care
Centre for Bioethics
Clinical Research Institute of Montreal
**www.ircm.qc.ca/bioethique/english/publications/
journal_of_palliative_care.html**

Academic journal covering the practical, critical thought on palliative care and palliative medicine.

Subscription required.

End-of-Life Care
American Medical Association (AMA)
www.ama-assn.org/ama/pub/category/2732.html

Click "End-of-Life Care" for professional resources.

Free to use.

End-of-Life Issues
Medline Plus
National Library of Medicine (NLM)
www.nlm.nih.gov/medlineplus/endoflifeissues.html

Extensive link resources. User must search links.

Free to use.

En Español ✐

Done Vida
www.donevida.org

Living Bank
www.livingbank.org
   Vaya → en Español

**Centros para el Control y la Prevención
de Enfermedades (CDC)**
www.cdc.gov/spanish

**NOAH—Acceso Computarizado a la Salud
de Nueva York**
www.noah-health.org/es/search/health.html

HON: Fundación Health on the Net
www.hon.ch/index_sp.html

Healthfinder Español
www.healthfinder.gov/espanol

**La Academia Estadounidense de Médicos
de Familia (AAFP)**
http://familydoctor.org/online/famdoces/home.html

Manual Merck de Informatión Médica
www.msd.es/publicaciones/mmerck_hogar/index.html

Medline Plus
Información de Salud para Usted
http://medlineplus.gov/spanish

Gobierno USA
www.usa.gov/gobiernousa/index.shtml

Salud de los Hispanoamericanos
Medline Plus
www.nlm.nih.gov/medlineplus/spanish/hispanic
americanhealth.html

Institutos Nacionales de la Salud (NIH)
http://salud.nih.gov

Información de Cáncer en Español
Instituto Nacional del Cáncer (NCI)
http://cancernet.nci.nih.gov/espanol

Instituto Nacional de Trastornos Neurológicos
y Accidentes Cerebrovascular (NINDS)
www.ninds.nih.gov/disorders/spanish/index.htm

El Instituto Nacional de la Salud Mental (NIMH)
www.nimh.nih.gov/publicat/pubListing.cfm?
pubType=spanish

Instituto Nacional de Artritis y Enfermedades Musculoesqueléticas y de la Piel (NIAMS)
www.niams.nih.gov/index_espanol.htm

Instituto Nacional de las Drogas de Abuso (NIDA)
www.nida.nih.gov/NIDAEspanol.html

Instituto Nacional del Ojo (NEI)
www.nei.nih.gov/health/espanol

Instituto Nacional de Imágenes Biomédicas y Biogenieria (NIBIB)
www.nibib.nih.gov/EnEspanol

Instituto Nacional de Investigación Dental y Craneofacial (NIDCR)
www.nidcr.nih.gov/espanol

Centro Coordinador Nacional de Información Sobre Enfermedades de los Riñones y de las Urinarias (NKUDIC)
http://kidney.niddk.nih.gov/spanish/indexsp.asp

Instituto Nacional de la Salud de Environmental (NIEHS)
www.niehs.nih.gov/external/espanol/home.htm

Instituto Nacional de Ciecias Médicas Generales
http://publications.nigms.nih.gov/espanol/pubs

La Administración de Drogas y Alimentos
de los Estados Unidos
www.fda.gov/oc/spanish/default.htm

La Salud Cardiovascular
American Heart Association (AHA)
www.americanheart.org/presenter.jhtml?
identifier=3015971

Organización Mundial de la Salud (WHO)
www.who.int/es/index.html

Enfermedades del Asma, Tabaco, Pulmón
American Lung Association (ALA)
www.lungusa.org/site/pp.asp?c=dvLUK9O0E&b=33214

La Diabetes y los Latinos
American Diabetes Association (ADA)
www.diabetes.org
    Vaya → en Español

Diccionario de la Diabetes (NIDDK)
http://diabetes.niddk.nih.gov/spanish/pubs/dictionary/
index.htm

Información en Español—Diabetes (NIDDK)
http://diabetes.niddk.nih.gov/spanish/indexsp.asp

Centro Nacional de Diseminación de Información Para Niños con Discapacidades (NICHCY)
http://nichcy.org/spanish.htm

Anomalías Congenitas—Genética y Teratología Sistemas Internacionales de Informacíon
http://ibis-birthdefects.org/start/spanish/index.htm

Inmunización Centros para el Control y la Prevención de Enfermedades (CDC)
www.cdc.gov/spanish/inmunizacion.htm

Inmunización Immunization Action Coalition (IAC)
www.immunize.org/catg.d/noneng.htm#spanish

Centro Nacional de Información Sobre la Salud de la Mujer
www.4woman.gov/espanol

OBGYN.net Latina
http://latina.obgyn.net/espanol

Reproline
Linea de Salud Repoductiva
www.reproline.jhu.edu/spanish/index.htm

Cáncer de Seno
La Universidad de Wisconsin—Madison
https://chess.chsra.wisc.edu/espanol/Home/
Home.aspx

Acción el Cáncer del Seno
www.bcaction.org
>   Vaya → en Español

Prevención del VIH/SIDA
Centros para el Control y la Prevención
Enfermedades (CDC)
www.cdc.gov/hiv/spanish/links.htm#resources

VIH/SIDA
AEGIS
www.aegis.com
>   Vaya → en Español.

Tutoriales Interactivos de Salud
Medline Plus
Información de Salud para usted
www.nlm.nih.gov/medlineplus/spanish/tutorial.html

InfoDoctor
www.infodoctor.org

Biblioteca Virtual en Salud
www.virtualhealthlibrary.org
Vaya → los Países de Latinoamerica y Europa

Latin America Network Information Center
Salud y Ciencias Médicas
http://lanic.utexas.edu/la/region/health

La Biblioteca Cochrane Plus
www.update-software.com/clibplus/clibplus.asp

Las Enfermedades Raras
www.kumc.edu/gec/support/spanish.html

LOLA
Organización Latina para Crear Conciencia Sobre el Hígado
www.lola-national.org/index_s.htm

Biblioteca Vitrual de Salud para Desastres
Organización Munidial de la Salud (WHO)
http://www.who.int/topics/diasters/es

La Medicina Complementaria y Alternativa
NOAH
www.noah-health.org/es/alternative

Harrison Online en Español
The McGraw-Hill Companies
a) www.harrisonmedicina.com
b) www.mcgraw-hill.com.mx
   Vaya → los Países de Latinoamerica y Europa

Actas de Medicina Gratis en Español
www.freemedicaljournals.com/htm/esp.htm

La Salud—Adolescentes y Mujeres
Cedar River Clinics—Seattle, Washington
www.fwhc.org/espanol/index.htm

Patología Pulmonar Inducida por Medicamentos
PneumoTox Online
www.pneumotox.com/index.php?lg=sp&nf=

Directrices Anticipadas y Órdenes de No Resucitar
La Academia Estadounidense de Médicos
de Familia (AAFP)
http://familydoctor.org/e003.xml

Información para Padres—Los Niños
Nemours Foundation
www.kidshealth.org/parent/en_espanol

Lesiones de la Médula Espinal
Instituto Caren Rehabilitacion Neurológica—
Buenos Aires, Argentina
www.neurorehabilitacion.com/trauma_medular.htm

Las Lesiones de la Médula Espina
Universidad de Virginia—Charlottesville, Virginia
www.healthsystem.virginia.edu/UVAHealth/
adult_pmr_sp/spcrd.cfm

Lesiones de la Médula Espina
Medline Plus
Información de Salud para Usted
www.nlm.nih.gov/medlineplus/spanish/tutorials/
spinalcordinjuryspanish/htm/index.htm

Atlas de Oftalmología
www.atlasophthalmology.com/atlas/text.jsf?locale=es

OncoLink—Tipos de Cancer La Universidad de Pensilvania
http://es.oncolink.org/types/es_index.cfm

Algoritmos Médicos
www.medal.org/visitor/www/spanish/index.html

Together Rx Access
www.togetherrxaccess.com/esp/home.html

Partnership for Prescription Assistance
www.pparx.org/intro.php
   Vaya → en Español

Medicare
www.medicare.gov/spanish/overview.asp

AARP en Español
www.aarp.org/espanol/

Erectile Dysfunction (ED)/ Impotence ✍

Erectile Dysfunction
eMedicine
www.emedicine.com/med/topic3023.htm
    Academic review of ED with other resources.
    Free to use.

Erectile Dysfunction
Medline Plus
National Library of Medicine (NLM)
www.nlm.nih.gov/medlineplus/erectiledysfunction.html
    Good general resource.
    Free to use.

Erectile Dysfunction
Medscape
www.medscape.com/resource/erectiledys
    Good general resource.
    Registration required.

Erectile Dysfunction
The New England Journal of Medicine (*NEJM*), 2000
Tom F. Lue, MD
http://content.nejm.org/cgi/content/short/342/24/1802

Academic review of ED.

Register, purchase, or subscribe.

"Erectile Dysfunction and Vascular Disease"
Postgraduate Medicine, 2003
Luciano Kolodny, MD
www.postgradmed.com/issues/2003/10_03/kolodny.htm

Good clinical review.

Free to use.

Evidence-Based Medicine (EBM) ᪄

Trip Database
Turning Research into Practice
www.tripdatabase.com:80/index.html
> Search database for EBM resources.
> Free to use.

Evidence-based Medicine
Hayward Medical Communications
www.evidence-based-medicine.co.uk/default.html
> Journals about evidence-based medicine.
> Subscription required for printed journals. Internet materials are free.

Cochrane
The Cochrane Collaboration
www.cochrane.org
> Collection of EBM databases.
> Free to use abstracts; full text requires subscription.

Centre for Evidence-Based Medicine—
Oxford, United Kingdom
www.cebm.net/index.asp
> EBM resources.
> Free to use.

Evidence-Based Medicine
Library of Health Sciences Peoria
University of Illinois—Chicago
www.uic.edu/depts/lib/lhsp/resources/ebm.shtml

Library search helping to find the best clinical literature.

Free to use.

Evidence-Based Practice
Health Links
University of Washington—Seattle, Washington
http://healthlinks.washington.edu/ebp

Great collection of EBM links.

Free to use, but some may require registration or subscription.

Evidence-Based Medicine
Karolinska Institutet—Stockholm, Sweden
www.mic.ki.se/EBM.html

Search extensive links.

Free to use.

Family Practice ✐

American Family Physician
American Academy of Family Physicians.
www.aafp.org/online/en/home.html
> Excellent professional journal.
> Subscription may be required.

Annals of Family Medicine
www.annfammed.org
> Professional journal covering Family Medicine.
> Free to use.

Merck Manual of Diagnosis and Therapy
www.merck.com/mmpe/index.html
> The eighteenth edition is available in print and Web versions.
> Purchase may be required.

BMJ Clinical Evidence
www.clinicalevidence.com/ceweb/conditions/index.jsp
> Extensive clinical resources.
> Subscription required.

Family Practice Notebook
www.fpnotebook.com
> An excellent Family Medicine resource.
> Free to use, but a subscription option is available.

General Practice Notebook
www.gpnotebook.co.uk/homePage.cfm

An online encyclopedia for family medicine practitioners from the United Kingdom.

Registration and purchases required.

Familydoctor.org
American Academy of Family Physicians
http://familydoctor.org/online/famdocen/home.html

Extensive health information for patients.

Free to use.

Gastroenterology/Abdominal Disorders ✒

Gastroenterology Journal Watch
http://gastroenterology.jwatch.org
GI (Gastroenterology) literature review.
Subscription required.

Gastroenterology
www.gastrojournal.org
Official journal of the American Gastroenterological Association Institute.
Subscription required.

Diagnostic Liver Pathology
Transplant Pathology Internet Services
Randall G. Lee, MD
http://tpis.upmc.edu
Academic liver pathology review.
Free to use.

Atlas of Gastrointestinal Endoscopy
www.endoatlas.com
Over 1,000 endoscopic images.
Free to use.

Gastroenterology
BioMed Central
www.biomedcentral.com/bmcgastroenterol
> Open access journal covering gastrointestinal disease.
> Free to use.

Viral Hepatitis
National Center for HIV/AIDS, STD, and TB Prevention
Centers for Disease Control and Prevention (CDC)
www.cdc.gov/ncidod/diseases/hepatitis/index.htm
> Comprehensive viral hepatitis resource.
> Free to use.

American Association for the Study of Liver Diseases
www.aasld.org/eweb/StartPage.aspx
> Use "Guidelines" for comprehensive literature review of liver diseases. Adobe Acrobat Reader is required.
> Free to use.

Gastroenterology
eMedicine
www.emedicine.com/med/GASTROENTEROLOGY.htm
> Extensive academic resource on gastrointestinal disease.
> Free to use.

Genetics/Genes/Heredity ∞

Bioinformatics and Genomics Gateway
BioMed Central
www.biomedcentral.com/gateways/bioinformaticsgenomics
    Online journal for genetics.
    Free to use.

National Human Genome Research Institute
National Institutes of Health (NIH)
www.genome.gov
    Extensive human genetics resources.
    Free to use.

American Journal of Human Genetics
The University of Chicago Press for The American Society for Human Genetics
www.journals.uchicago.edu/AJHG
    Academic journal for human genetics.
    Subscription required.

American Journal of Medical Genetics
John Wiley & Sons, Inc.
www3.interscience.wiley.com/cgi-bin/jhome/33129
    Academic journal for medical genetics.
    Subscription required.

Annual Review of Genetics
Annual Reviews, Inc.
http://arjournals.annualreviews.org/loi/genet?cookieset=1
> Academic genetics journal.
> Subscription required.

Cancer Chromosomes
National Center for Biotechnology Information (NCBI)
www.ncbi.nlm.nih.gov/entrez/query.fcgi?
db=cancerchromosomes
> Cancer database for cytogenetic, clinical, and reference information.
> Registration required.

Genes and Disease
National Center for Biotechnology Information (NCBI)
www.ncbi.nlm.nih.gov/books/bv.fcgi?call=bv.View.
ShowTOC&rid=gnd.TOC&depth=2
> Disease-oriented database reviewing genetics.
> Free to use.

Genetics in Medicine
Lippincott Williams & Wilkins
www.geneticsinmedicine.org
> Official journal of the American College of Medical Genetics.
> Subscription required.

Genomics and Health Weekly Update
Centers for Disease Control and Prevention (CDC)
www.cdc.gov/genomics/update/current.htm
> Resources on the impact of human genetic disease.
> Free to use.

HumGen International

www.humgen.umontreal.ca/int/index.cfm?lang=1

International database of legal, social, and ethics of human genetics. Also, French and Spanish versions are available.

Free to use.

National Center for Biotechnology Information (NCBI)
National Library of Medicine (NLM)

www.ncbi.nlm.nih.gov

Comprehensive national resource for molecular biology information.

Free to use.

Influenza Genome Sequencing Project
National Institute of Allergy and Infectious
Diseases (NIAID)
National Institutes of Health (NIH)

www.niaid.nih.gov/dmid/genomes/mscs/influenza.htm

Comprehensive database covering the genome knowledge base of influenza.

Free to use.

Gene Tests
University of Washington—Seattle, Washington

www.genetests.org

Extensive genetics information resource. Search "GeneReviews."

Free to use.

Geriatrics/Old Age/Aging ∾

Geriatrics
BioMed Central
www.biomedcentral.com/bmcgeriatr
> Open access journal on geriatrics.
> Free to use.

Geriatrics and Aging
www.geriatricsandaging.ca/
> Provides education about health concerns of older adults.
> Free to access some information. Subscription required for the journal.

The American Geriatrics Society
www.americangeriatrics.org
> Professional society dedicated to the health of older Americans.
> Some educational materials require a fee.

The Merck Manual of Geriatrics
www.merck.com/mkgr/mmg/home.jsp
> Academic review of geriatrics.
> Online version is free.

NIHSeniorHealth.gov
http://nihseniorhealth.gov
Government site for geriatrics.
Free to use.

Geriatric Care
Medscape
www.medscape.com/resource/geriatric
Thorough geriatric resources.
Registration required.

Administration on Aging (AOA)
U.S. Department of Health and Human Services
www.aoa.gov
Comprehensive geriatric resources for professionals, patients, and family members.
Free to use.

National Clearinghouse for Long-Term Care Information
U.S. Department of Health and Human Services
www.longtermcare.gov
Extensive resources on long-term care.
Free to use.

Ageline Database
American Association of Retired Persons (AARP)
www.aarp.org/research/ageline
Extensive geriatric resource.
Free to use.

Headaches ✑

Headache Information Page
National Institute of Neurological Disorders and
Stroke (NINDS)
National Institutes of Health (NIH)
www.ninds.nih.gov/disorders/headache/headache.htm
> General information resource site.
> Free to use.

Headache
Family Practice Notebook
www.fpnotebook.com/NEUCh15.htm
> Family practice headache overview.
> Free to use, but a subscription option is available.

Headache
Medline Plus
National Library of Medicine (NLM)
www.nlm.nih.gov/medlineplus/headache.html
> General headache information references.
> Free to use.

Headache
Medscape
www.medscape.com/resource/headache
Thorough clinical and research headache review.
Registration required.

The Facts About Headaches
HealthLink
Medical College of Wisconsin—Milwaukee, Wisconsin
http://healthlink.mcw.edu/article/946414636.html
Brief but factual headache review.
Free to use.

Headache, Migraine
eMedicine
www.emedicine.com/emerg/topic230.htm
Excellent clinical review of migraine headaches plus other
headache resources.
Free to use.

Migraine and Headache
Bandolier
www.jr2.ox.ac.uk/bandolier/booth/booths/migraine.html
Evidence-based literature review for migraine headaches and
other headache conditions.
Subscription required for access to articles.

American Headache Society
www.americanheadachesociety.org
Professional society dedicated to the study and treatment of
headache and face pain. Review "Professional Resources."
Free to use.

National Headache Foundation
www.headaches.org
> Review "Healthcare Professionals" for headache resources.
> Free to use.

Pediatric Headache
Neurology
www.neurology.org/cgi/collection/pediatric_headache
> Pediatric literature review of headaches with listing of other
> pediatric-related headache conditions.
> Subscription required for article access.

"Headaches in Children and Adolescents"
American Family Physician, 2002
Donald W. Lewis, MD
www.aafp.org/afp/20020215/625.html
> Headache review for children.
> Free to use.

"Practice Parameter: Evaluation of Children and Adolescents with Recurrent Headaches"
Neurology, 2002
www.neurology.org/cgi/reprint/59/4/490.pdf
> Clinical practice guidelines for children with headaches.
> Free to use.

Headaches in Children
Family Practice Notebook
www.fpnotebook.com/NEU185.htm
> Thorough primary care review of pediatric headaches.
> Free to use, but subscription option is available.

Pediatric Headache
eMedicine

a.) Migraine Headache: Pediatric Perspective
www.emedicine.com/neuro/topic529.htm

b.) Childhood Migraine Variants
www.emedicine.com/neuro/topic494.htm

c.) Headache, Children
www.emedicine.com/oph/topic334.htm

d.) Pediatrics, Headache
www.emedicine.com/emerg/topic382.htm

e.) Headache: Pediatric Perspective
www.emedicine.com/NEURO/topic528.htm

Thorough clinical reviews of pediatric headaches with other clinical resources.

Free to use.

Health Care Policy ✏

National Health Policy Forum
The George Washington University—Washington, DC
www.nhpf.org
   Excellent resource on health policy primarily for senior congressional staff, the executive branch and congressional support agencies.
   Free to use.

Duke Health Policy Gateway
Center for Health Policy, Law, and Management
Duke University—Durham, North Carolina
www.hpolicy.duke.edu/cyberexchange
   Excellent and comprehensive database.
   Free to use.

Duke Center for Clinical Health Policy Research
Duke University—Durham, North Carolina
http://clinpol.mc.duke.edu/main
   Excellent resource. Review "Evidence-Based Practice Center, Disease Modeling and Implementation."
   Free to use.

Health Policy Monitor
www.hpm.org/index.jsp
>An international network for health policy and reform.
>Free to use.

The Library of Congress
Thomas
http://thomas.loc.gov
>Search for health care policy legislative information from the
>Library of Congress.
>Free to use.

Health Resource Policy and Systems
BioMed Central
www.health-policy-systems.com
>An online journal devoted to health care policy.
>Free to use.

Health Affairs: The Policy Journal of the Health Sphere
http://healthaffairs.org
>Comprehensive journal reviewing health care policy.
>Subscription required.

The Campaign for Mental Health Reform
www.mhreform.org
>Mental health care policy and reform.
>Free to use.

State Cancer Legislative Database Program
National Cancer Institute (NCI)
http://scld-nci.net

Database of state cancer-related legislation covering breast cancer, colorectal cancer, prostate cancer, tobacco, treatments, and more.

Free to use.

National Academy for State Health Policy
www.nashp.org

Access to resources helping states achieve excellence in state health policy and practice.

Free to use.

Center for Health Services Research and Policy
The George Washington University Center for Health Services Research and Policy—Washington, DC
www.gwumc.edu/sphhs/healthpolicy/chsrp

Excellent "links" to resources. User must search links.

Free to use.

Center for Health and Public Policy Studies
University of California—Berkeley, California
School of Public Health
http://chpps.berkeley.edu

Research and policy analysis in health policy/politics for California and the nation. Excellent "Links" resource.

Free to use.

Hematology/Blood Disorders ∽

Bloodline
www.bloodline.net
The online resource for hematology education and news.
Free to use.

Platelets on the Internet
James N. George, MD
University of Oklahoma College of Medicine—
Oklahoma City, Oklahoma
http://moon.ouhsc.edu/jgeorge
Review of ITP (Idiopathic Thrombocytopenia Purpura), TTP
(Thrombotic Thrombocytopenia Purpura), HUS (Hemolytic Uremic
Syndrome) and DIT (Drug-Induced Thrombocytopenia).
Free to use.

Current Opinion in Hematology
Lippincott Williams & Wilkins
www.co-hematology.com
Academic hematology journal.
Subscription required.

HemostasisCME.org
www.hemostasiscme.org
Educational resource on hemostasis management.
Free to use.

Atlas of Hematology
Nivaldo Medeiros, MD
São Paulo, Brazil
www.hematologyatlas.com
> Extensive hematologic images.
> Free to use.

Hematology
eMedicine
www.emedicine.com/med/Hematology.htm
> Extensive academic resources.
> Free to use.

American Journal of Hematology
John Wiley & Sons, Inc.
www3.interscience.wiley.com/cgi-bin/jhome/35105/
> Academic hematology journal.
> Subscription required.

Karolinska Institutet
Stockholm, Sweden
www.mic.ki.se/Diseases/c15.html
> Extensive listing of blood diseases. User must search links.
> Free to use.

Hematopathology Index
http://library.med.utah.edu/WebPath/HEMEHTML/
HEMEIDX.html
> Review blood smears on "Standard Peripheral Blood and Marrow
> Findings," "RBC and Bone Marrow Disorders," and "Leukemias."
> Free to use.

High-Altitude Medicine ∾

High-Altitude Medicine Guide
Thomas E. Dietz, MD
www.high-altitude-medicine.com
> Current academic information on altitude illness and more.
> Free to use.

High-Altitude Medicine and Biology
Mary Ann Liebert, Inc.
www.liebertpub.com/publication.aspx?pub_id=65
> Academic journal covering high-altitude life sciences.
> Subscription required.

British Mountaineering Council
UIAA Mountain Medicine Centre
www.thebmc.co.uk/feature.aspx?id=1921
> Extensive clinical infomation and related topics.
> Free to use.

Altitude Illness—Pulmonary Syndromes
eMedicine
www.emedicine.com/emerg/topic795.htm
> Excellent clinical review article.
> Free to use.

Pulmonary Edema, High Altitude
eMedicine
www.emedicine.com/med/topic1956.htm
> Excellent clinical review article.
> Free to use.

High-Altitude Medicine and Physiology, 3rd edition, 2001
M. P. Ward, J. S. Milledge, and J. B. West
http://thorax.bmjjournals.com/cgi/content/full/56/7/586
> Book review for the standard textbook on high-altitude medicine.
> Purchase required.

Everest BC Clinic 5500m
www.basecampmd.com
> Review multiple topics in the "Guide to High-Altitude Medicine."
> Free to use.

Hyperlipidemia/High Blood Lipids/Cholesterol ∽

Lipid Resource Center
eMedicine
www.emedicine.com/rc/rc/i1/lipid.htm
> Excellent academic/clinical resource covering lipid disorders.
> Free to use.

Hyperlipidemia
Medscape
www.medscape.com/resource/hyperlipidemia
> Excellent clinical resource covering all aspects of hyperlipidemia.
> Registration required.

Detection, Evaluation, and Treatment of High Blood Cholesterol in Adults
Adult Treatment Panel lll, 2005
National Heart, Lung, and Blood Institute (NHLBI)
www.nhlbi.nih.gov/guidelines/cholesterol
> National guidelines for the treatment of high blood cholesterol.
> Free to use.

Hyperlipidemia
Family Practice Notebook
www.fpnotebook.com/CVCh12.htm

General medical practice review of high blood lipids.

Free to use, but subscription option is available.

National Lipid Association
www.lipid.org

Excellent resource. Review "Clinical Articles," "Education," and more.

Mostly free, but membership required for certain aspects.

The Cholesterol LOW DOWN
American Heart Association (AHA)
www.cholesterollowdown.org/Footer/For_Healthcare_ Professionals.html

Very useful information regarding cholesterol.

Free to use.

CVspectrum.org
www.cvspectrum.org

A comprehensive dyslipidemic and atherosclerosis resource.

Registration required.

When Should We Screen Children for Hyperlipidemia?
University of Washington Health Sciences Library
http://healthlinks.washington.edu/hsl/liaisons/stanna/ fpin/hyperlipidemia

Excellent links covering children and lipid disorders.

Some resources may have access restrictions.

Hypertension/High Blood Pressure ✑

"The Seventh Report of the Joint National Committee on Prevention, Detection, Evaluation, and Treatment of High Blood Pressure (JNC-7)"
National Institutes of Health (NIH)
www.nhlbi.nih.gov/guidelines/hypertension/index.htm

National guidelines for high blood pressure.

Free to use.

Hypertension
eMedicine

www.emedicine.com/med/topic1106.htm

Thorough academic review of hypertension.

Free to use.

Hypertensive Heart Disease
eMedicine

www.emedicine.com/med/topic3432.htm

Academic review of high blood pressure and the heart.

Free to use.

High Blood Pressure
Medline Plus
National Library of Medicine (NLM)
www.nlm.nih.gov/medlineplus/highbloodpressure.html
> Thorough collection covering high blood pressure resources.
> Free to use.

Lowering Your Blood Pressure with DASH
(Dietary Approaches to Stop Hypertension)
National Heart, Lung, and Blood Institute (NHLBI)
www.nhlbi.nih.gov/health/public/heart/hbp/dash
> Dietary guidelines for blood-pressure reduction.
> Free to use.

Hypertension
Journal Watch
www.jwatch.org/cgi/collection/hypertension
> Journal article collection reviewing hypertension.
> Subscription required.

Resistant or Difficult-to-Control Hypertension
The New England Journal of Medicine (*NEJM*), 2006
Clinical Practice
Marvin Moser, MD, et al
http://content.nejm.org/cgi/content/short/355/4/385
> A clinical vignette highlighting hypertension.
> Register, purchase, or subscribe.

Hypertension
Lippincott Williams & Wilkins/American Heart Association
http://hyper.ahajournals.org
Professional journal reviewing hypertension.
Subscription required.

American Journal of Hypertension
Elsevier
www.ajh-us.org
Professional journal for hypertension and heart disease.
Subscription required.

Hypertension Online
Baylor College of Medicine—Houston, Texas
www.hypertensiononline.org
Educational site for hypertension.
Free to use.

Infection Control ✑

Infection Control Department
University of California—San Francisco, California
http://infectioncontrol.ucsfmedicalcenter.org
   Comprehensive resource materials for hospital epidemiology and infection control at UCSF Medical Center.
   Free to use.

Hospital Epidemiology and Infection Control
Johns Hopkins Medicine—Baltimore, Maryland
www.hopkinsmedicine.org/heic
   Great clinical resource for Infectious Diseases, Occupational Health, Bioterrorism, Pandemic Influenza, MRSA, and more.
   Free to use.

Infection Control in Health Care Settings
Centers for Disease Control and Prevention (CDC)
www.cdc.gov/ncidod/dhqp/index.html
   Fantastic resource covering Healthcare-Associated Infections, Protecting Patients, Protecting Healthcare Workers, Infection Control Guidelines and more.
   Free to use.

American Journal of Infection Control
Elsevier
www.us.elsevierhealth.com/product.jsp?isbn=01966553
Published by Elsevier for the Association for Professionals in Infection Control and Epidemiology, Inc.
Subscription required.

Association for Professionals in Infection Control and Epidemiology
www.apic.org
Review "Education," "Government Advocacy," "Practice Guidance," and "Publications."
Mostly free materials.

National Resource for Infection Control
www.nric.org.uk
A UK-based resource for up-to-date evidence-based information in infection control.
Free to use.

The Society for the Healthcare Epidemiology in America (SHEA)
www.shea-online.org
Professional society for the advancement of the science of health care epidemiology.
Free materials available, and membership required access.

Infectious Diseases (ID) ✑

Centers for Disease Control and Prevention (CDC)
U.S. Department of Health and Human Services
www.cdc.gov
> Extensive resources.
> Free to use.

Morbidity and Mortality Weekly Review (MMWR)
www.cdc.gov/mmwr
> Excellent CDC publication reviewing worldwide infectious
diseases.
> Free to use.

National Center for Infectious Diseases
Centers for Disease Control and Prevention (CDC)
www.cdc.gov/ncidod/index.htm
> Excellent comprehensive ID resource.
> Free to use.

The ABX Guide
Johns Hopkins University, Division of Infectious
Diseases—Baltimore, Maryland
http://hopkins-abxguide.org
> Comprehensive antibiotic guide.
> Free download version, but purchase required for print version.

Emerging Infectious Diseases
National Institutes of Health (NIH)
The Division of Microbiology and Infectious Diseases
**www3.niaid.nih.gov/healthscience/healthtopics/emerging/
default.htm**
> Extensive resources.
> Free to use.

National Institute of Allergy and Infectious Diseases
National Institutes of Health (NIH)
www3.niaid.nih.gov
> Extensive clinical resources.
> Free to use.

The Sanford Guide
www.sanfordguide.com
> Comprehensive antimicrobial guide.
> Purchase required.

National Foundation for Infectious Diseases
www.nfid.org
> Educating health care professionals about the causes, treatment,
and prevention of infectious diseases.
> Free to use and purchases available.

Infectious Diseases in Children
SLACK, Inc.
www.idinchildren.com
> Pediatric ID publication.
> Registration and/or subscription required.

Sepsis.com
Eli Lily and Company
www.sepsis.com
> Clinical review of sepsis.
> Free to use.

JAMA Bioterrorism
http://jama.ama-assn.org/cgi/collection/bioterrorism
> Collection of bioterrorism articles.
> Subscription or article purchase required.

Disease Outbreak News
Epidemic and Pandemic Alert and Response (EPR)
World Health Organization (WHO)
www.who.int/csr/don/en
> Latest information on disease outbreaks.
> Free to use.

Infections Diseases
eMedicine
a.) Internal Medicine
> **www.emedicine.com/med/INFECTIOUS_
> DISEASES.htm**

b.) Pediatrics
> **www.emedicine.com/ped/INFECTIOUS_
> DISEASES.htm.**

> Thorough clinical reviews of ID.
> Free to use.

Internal Medicine/ Adult Medicine ✒

Access Medicine
McGraw-Hill Companies
www.accessmedicine.com
> Extensive medical resources.
> Subscription required.

MDChoice.com
www.mdchoice.com
> "The ultimate medical information finder."
> Free to use.

American College of Physician Guidelines
www.acponline.org/clinical/guidelines/?in
> Comprehensive clinical practice guidelines.
> Free to use.

Disease Management Project
The Cleveland Clinic
www.clevelandclinicmeded.com/diseasemanagement

Review the following: "Allergy and Immunology," "Cardiology," "Dermatology," "Endocrine," "Gastroenterology and Hepatology," "Hematology and Oncology," "Infections Diseases," "Nephrology," "Neurology," "Psychiatry," "Pulmonary," "Rheumatology," and "Women's Health."

Free to use, but a fee is required for Continuing Medical Education.

Journals ⤷

Free Medical Journals
www.freemedicaljournals.com
   Access to online, free, and full-text journals.
   Free to use.

Amedeo: The Medical Literature Guide
www.amedeo.com
   Search the literature by medical specialty or topic.

Ovid
www.ovid.com/site/index.jsp
   "Access the latest, most trusted scientific medical and academic
   research journals."

The New England Journal of Medicine
http://content.nejm.org

Annals of Internal Medicine
www.annals.org

The Journal of the American Medical Association (JAMA)
http://jama.ama-assn.org

Archives of Internal Medicine
http://archinte.ama-assn.org

Medicine
www.md-journal.com

The Lancet
www.thelancet.com

Mayo Clinic Proceedings
www.mayoclinicproceedings.com

Annual Reviews
Intelligent Synthesis of the Scientific Literature
http://www.annualreviews.org

Library of the National Medical Society
www.medical-library.org

Medical-Journals.com
www.medical-journals.com

Merck Medicus
www.merckmedicus.com/pp/us/hcp/templates/tier3/
journals.jsp

The Clinics of North America
www.theclinics.com

Search the journal abstracts free. Free journals may be six to twelve months old. Register, purchase, or subscribe.

Lung Cancer &

National Cancer Institute (NCI)
National Institutes of Health (NIH)
www.cancer.gov/cancertopics/types/lung
　　Review "PDQ," "Treatment," "Prevention," "Screening," and much more clinical information.
　　Free to use.

Lung Cancers
OncoLink
Abramson Cancer Center of the University of Pennsylvania—Philadelphia, Pennsylvania
www.oncolink.org/types/types.cfm?c=9
　　Review "Lung Cancer," "Mesothelioma," "Non-Small Cell Lung Cancer," "Small-Cell Lung Cancer," plus additional clinical resources.
　　Free to use.

Lung Cancer
MedLine Plus
National Library of Medicine (NLM)
www.nlm.nih.gov/medlineplus/lungcancer.html
　　Thorough general references on lung cancer.
　　Free to use.

Lung Cancer
Medscape
www.medscape.com/resource/lungcancer
Good clinical content reviewing lung cancer.
Registration required.

Facts About Lung Cancer
American Lung Association (ALA)
www.lungusa.org/site/pp.asp?c=dvLUK9OOE&b=35427
General fact sheet reviewing important concepts on lung cancer.
Free to use.

Lung Cancer
Centers for Disease Control and Prevention (CDC)
www.cdc.gov/cancer/lung
Good general lung cancer resource. Review "Quick Links" and
"Cancer Burden."
Free to use.

American Society of Clinical Oncology (ASCO)
http://lungca.asco.org
Review academic resources covering all aspects of lung cancer.
Subscription may be required.

Lung Cancer, Non-Small Cell
eMedicine
www.emedicine.com/med/topic1333.htm
Thorough review of lung cancer with other related clinical topics.
Free to use.

Lung Cancer Online Foundation
www.lungcanceronline.org

Good clinical resources for patients and family members. Review clinical topic sections.

Free to use.

"Lung Cancer in U. S. Women: A Contemporary Epidemic"
The Journal of the American Medical Association (JAMA)
Jyoti D. Patel, MD, et al, 2004
http://jama.ama-assn.org/cgi/content/abstract/291/14/1763

Good clinical review of women and lung cancer, plus the site allows access to other related lung cancer articles.

Subscription required.

"Lung Cancer and the Sexes"
Time Magazine, 2006
Christine Gorman
www.time.com/time/magazine/article/0,9171,1214947,00.html

Review lung cancer differences between women and men.

Free to use.

"Lung Cancer Immunotherapy"
Clinical Medicine and Research, 2005
Luis E. Raez, MD, et al
www.pubmedcentral.nih.gov/articlerender.fcgi?artid=1288407

Review of antitumor (antibody) immunotherapy for lung cancer.

Free to use.

"Survival of Patients with Stage I Lung Cancer Detected on CT Screening"
The Interventional Early Lung Cancer Action Program Investigators
The New England Journal of Medicine (*NEJM*), 2006
http://content.nejm.org/cgi/content/short/355/17/1763

Discussion of lung cancer screening and its findings with Stage I disease.

Register, purchase, or subscribe.

International Early Lung Cancer Action Program (I-ELCAP)
www.ielcap.org

Professional organization reviewing the need for early diagnosis, treatment, and cures for lung cancer.

Free to use.

Lung Cancer Screening
National Cancer Institute(NCI)
www.cancer.gov/cancertopics/pdq/screening/lung/ healthprofessionals

Academic review on lung cancer screening.

Free to use.

Medicare ✑

Medicare
U.S. Department of Health and Human Services
www.medicare.gov
> Comprehensive site for Medicare resources.
> Free to use.

Medicare
Medline Plus
National Library of Medicine (NLM)
www.nlm.nih.gov/medlineplus/medicare.html
> Extensive Medicare resources.
> Free to use.

Medicare Prescription Drug Plan
Medline Plus
National Library of Medicine (NLM)
www.nlm.nih.gov/medlineplus/medicareprescription
drugplan.html
> Extensive review of resources on Medicare prescription drug
> coverage.
> Free to use.

Medicare Prescription Drug Plan Resources
American Academy of Family Physicians
http://familydoctor.org/867.xml
   Listing of additional resources for Medicare Part D and more.
   Free to use.

Medicare
Prescription Drug Coverage
U.S. Department of Health and Human Services
www.medicare.gov/pdphome.asp
   Comprehensive resource.
   Free to use.

Medicare
Social Security Online
www.ssa.gov/mediinfo.htm
   Excellent resources.
   Free to use.

National Bipartisan Commission on the
Future of Medicare
http://medicare.commission.gov/medicare/index.html
   Extensive federal report on Medicare, its future, and current
legislation.
   Free to use.

Medicare
Public Agenda
www.publicagenda.org/issues/overview.cfm?
issue_type=medicare
   Thorough overview on Medicare and concerns regarding its survival.
   Free to use.

Medicare Central
Families USA
www.familiesusa.org/issues/medicare/medicare-central-home.html
> Consumer health care information on Medicare.
> Free to use.

Administration on Aging
U.S. Department of Health and Human Services
www.aoa.gov
> Excellent resources for older Americans with translations in German, Spanish, French, Italian, Korean, Japanese, Chinese, and Portuguese.
> Free to use.

Medicare Rights Center
www.medicarerights.org
> Your information guide through the Medicare maze.
> Free to use.

Menopause/Change of Life ∽

Menopause
eMedicine
www.emedicine.com/med/topic3289.htm

Excellent academic discussion. Review "Menopause Resource Center."

Free to use.

Menopause
Medscape
www.medscape.com/resource/menopause

Good collection of resources.

Registration required.

Menopause
Medline Plus
National Library of Medicine (NLM)
www.nlm.nih.gov/medlineplus/menopause.html

Excellent general resources.

Free to use.

Women's Reproductive Health: Menopause
Centers for Disease Control and Prevention (CDC)
www.cdc.gov/reproductivehealth//WomensRH/
Menopause.htm
Good resource and selected references.
Free to use.

Menopause and Perimenopause
OBGYN.net
www.obgyn.net/menopause
Thorough resources for menopause.
Mostly free materials.

Menopause Collection
JAMA and Archives Journals
http://pubs.ama-assn.org/cgi/collection/menopause_
Medical literature collection on menopause.
Subscription required.

Menopause (Incl HRT)
British Medical Journal Topic Collections
http://www.bmj.com/cgi/collection/menopause
Academic medical literature review.
Subscription required.

Neonatology/Newborn Disorders ✍

Neofax
http://neofax.com
> The premier neonatal drug reference manual.
> Purchase required.

Neonatology on the Web
www.neonatology.com
> Neonatal resources. Check "Clinical Resources."
> Free to use.

Neofix
David Clark, MD, Chairman of Pediatrics
Children's Hospital at Albany Medical Center—
Albany, New York
www.pedialink.org/pedialink/neopix/index2.cfm
> Neonatal images of diseases.
> Free to use.

Neonatal Handbook
Newborn Emergency Transport Services (NETS)
Victoria, Australia
www.netsvic.org.au/nets/handbook/index.cfm?doc_id=447
> Extensive clinical neonatal topics.
> Free to use.

Nephrology/Kidney Disorders ✑

National Kidney Foundation
www.kidney.org
   Review "Professionals" and "Transplantation" for clinical resources.
   Subscription and/or purchase may be required.

Hypertension, Dialysis, and Clinical Nephrology
www.hdcn.com
   Extensive academic resources.
   Registration, subscription, and/or purchase may be required.

Atlas of Renal Pathology
American Journal of Kidney Diseases (AJKD)
www2.us.elsevierhealth.com/ajkd/atlas
   Collection of renal pathology slides for teaching.
   Free to use, but AJKD requires a subscription.

CyberNephrology
www.cybernephrology.org
   Useful clinical information on adult and pediatric nephrology.
   Free to use, but some purchases required.

Nephrology Rounds
Nephrology Division
Brigham and Women's Hospital—Boston, Massachusetts
www.nephrologyrounds.org
Extensive academic resources.
Free to use.

Renal Pathology Tutorial
The Nephropathology Lab
University of North Carolina—Chapel Hill
www.uncnephropathology.org
Renal pathology review.
Free to use.

Nephrology Pharmacy Associates
www.nephrologypharmacy.com
Search "Publications" for educational materials on renal disease, Peritoneal Dialysis drug interactions, dialysis of drugs, and more.
Free to use.

Neurology/Brain, Spine, and Nerve Disorders ∾

The Internet Stroke Center
Stroke Center at Barnes-Jewish Hospital and Washington University School of Medicine—St. Louis, Missouri
www.strokecenter.org
Excellent academic resource on stroke reviewing types and symptoms, guidelines and consensus statements, assessment tools and stroke imaging.
Free to use.

CNS Diseases
Karolinska Institute—Stockholm, Sweden
www.mic.ki.se/Diseases/C10.228.html
Extensive neurology links organized by disease. User must search links.
Free to use.

Cerebrospinal Fluid Research
BioMed Central
www.cerebrospinalfluidresearch.com
Journal regarding CSF in health and disease.
Free to use.

Neurology
BioMed Central
www.biomedcentral.com/bmcneurol
> Online neurology journal.
> Free to use.

Neurology Case of the Month
Baylor College of Medicine—Houston, Texas
www.bcm.edu/neurol/case.html
> Interesting and challenging neurology case presentations.
> Free to use.

Interactive Brain Atlas
University of Washington—Seattle, Washington
John Sundsten
http://www9.biostr.washington.edu/da.html
> Great neuroanatomy resources.
> Free to use.

Neuroradiology Library
University of Iowa—Iowa City, Iowa
www.uiowa.edu/~c064s01
> Image collection of normal and central nervous system diseases.
> Free to use.

Neuroexam.com
www.neuroexam.com
> An interactive online guide to the Neurologic Exam.
> Free to use.

Neurology
Lippincott Williams & Wilkins
www.neurology.org
> Official journal of the American Academy of Neurology.
> Subscription required.

Neurosciences on the Internet
www.neuroguide.com
> Index of neuroscience resources.
> Free to use.

National Institute of Neurological Disorders and Stroke (NINDS)
www.ninds.nih.gov/index.htm
> Federal organization studying neurologic disease. Review "Disorder Index."
> Free to use.

American Stroke Association
www.strokeassociation.org/presenter.jhtml? identifier=3030388
> Review "For Health Care Professionals" and "Professional Resources."
> Free to use.

Neurology
eMedicine
www.emedicine.com/neuro/index.shtml
> Academic article collection on neurologic disease.
> Free to use.

Neurologic Exam
Paul D. Larsen, MD
University of Nebraska School of Medicine
Suzanne S. Stensaas, MD
University of Utah School of Medicine
http://library.med.utah.edu/neurologicexam/html/home_
exam.html

Clinical site for neurology exam. Review "Neurologic Cases" and "PediNeurologic Exam."

Free to use.

Neuromuscular Disease Center
Washington University—St. Louis, Missouri
www.neuro.wustl.edu/neuromuscular

Excellent academic site reviewing clinical and basic science information on neuromuscular disease.

Free to use.

MD Virtual University
WEMOVE
www.mdvu.org

Professionals' movement-disorder resource.

Free to use.

Neurosurgery/Brain and Spinal Cord Surgery ⸎

Neurosurgical Focus
Medscape
www.medscape.com/viewpublication/65_index
   Neurosurgical clinical and research topics reviewed.
   Registration required.

Neurosurgery: ON-CALL
www.neurosurgery.org
   Professional organization formed by the Congress of Neurological
Surgeons and the American Association of Neurological Surgeons.
Review "Neurosurgical Subspecialty Sections."
   Some materials are free; membership required.

Congress of Neurologic Surgeons
www.neurosurgeon.org
   Review "Education" section.
   Membership required, but some materials are free.

Neurosurgical Service
Massachusetts General Hospital
Harvard Medical School—Boston, Massachusetts
http://neurosurgery.mgh.harvard.edu/rounds/

Review "Education Links" and "Grand Rounds."

Free to use.

Neurology and Neurosurgey Grand Rounds
The University of Arizona Health Sciences
Center—Tucson, Arizona
http://video.biocom.arizona.edu/video/videolibrary/
NeuroGR/

Download clinical grand rounds presentations.

Free to use.

Neurosurgery
eMedicine
www.emedicine.com/med/NEUROSURGERY.htm

Academic article collection reviewing neurosurgery topics.

Free to use.

Nutrition ✌

Nutrition.gov
U.S. Department of Agriculture (USDA)
www.nutrition.gov
> Online access to government information on nutrition.
> Free to use.

Food and Nutrition Information Center (FNIC)
U.S. Department of Agriculture (USDA)
http://fnic.nal.usda.gov
> Extensive nutritional resources.
> Free to use.

My Pyramid
U.S. Department of Agriculture (USDA)
www.mypyramid.gov
> Resources to help improve nutrition, dietary guidance, and well-being of Americans.
> Free to use.

Center for Nutrition Policy and Promotion (CNPP)
U.S. Department of Agriculture (USDA)
www.cnpp.usda.gov
> Developing and promoting dietary guidance that links scientific research to nutritional needs.
> Free to use.

The Nutrition Source
Harvard School of Public Health—Boston, Massachusetts
www.hsph.harvard.edu/nutritionsource
> Extensive academic nutrition information.
> Free to use.

Nutrition
World Health Organization (WHO)
www.who.int/nutrition/en
> Global nutrition review and resources.
> Free to use.

Nutrition Journal
BioMed Central
www.nutritionj.com
> Online journal covering human/clinical nutrition and research.
> Free to use.

American Journal of Clinical Nutrition
The American Society for Nutrition
www.ajcn.org
> Academic nutrition journal.
> Subscription required.

Office of Dietary Supplements (ODS)
National Institutes of Health (NIH)
http://ods.od.nih.gov
> Excellent resource for dietary supplements.
> Free to use.

Center for Food Safety and Applied Nutrition
U.S. Food and Drug Administration (FDA)
www.cfsan.fda.gov
> Excellent nutrition resource.
> Free to use.

Nutritional and Metabolic Disorders
Karolinska Institutet—Stockholm, Sweden
www.mic.ki.se/Diseases/C18.html
> Extensive collection of links. User must search.
> Free to use.

The Blonz Guide
Edward Blonz, PhD, MS, FACN
http://blonz.com
> Extensive academic/educational links on nutrition, food, and
> health. User must search.
> Free to use.

The Center for Human Nutrition
The University of Texas
Southwestern Medical Center—Dallas, Texas
www.utsouthwestern.edu/utsw/cda/dept27712/files/
40245.html
> Excellent academic nutrition resource.
> Free to use.

Food and Nutrition Service
Nutrition Assistance Programs
U.S. Department of Agriculture(USDA)
www.fns.usda.gov/fns

Resource for nutritional assistance provided to children and low-income people.

Free to use.

Nutrition and Fitness
Kids Health
Nemours Foundation
www.kidshealth.org/parent/nutrition_fit/index.html

Good resource for parents on kids' nutrition and fitness.

Free to use.

Kids' Nutrition
Baylor College of Medicine—Houston, Texas
www.kidsnutrition.org

Good children's nutritional resource.

Free to use.

Child Nutrition
Medline Plus
National Library of Medicine (NLM)
www.nlm.nih.gov/medlineplus/childnutrition.html

Excellent child nutrition resource.

Free to use.

Clinical Nutrition
Children's Memorial Hospital—Chicago, Illinois
**www.childrensmemorial.org/depts/clinicalnutrition/
links.asp**

Excellent collection of pediatric nutrition links.

Free to use.

Obesity ∽

Overweight and Obesity
Centers for Disease Control and Prevention (CDC)
www.cdc.gov/nccdphp/dnpa/obesity
Obesity overview.
Free to use.

Weight-Control Information Network
Understanding Adult Obesity
National Institute of Diabetes and Digestive
and Kidney Disease (NIDDK)
http://win.niddk.nih.gov/publications/understanding.htm
Review of adult obesity.
Free to use.

Obesity Treatment Guidelines
National Heart, Lung, and Blood Institute (NHLBI)
www.nhlbi.nih.gov/guidelines/obesity/ob_home.htm
Clinical guidelines on overweight and obesity in adults.
Free, downloadable materials.

Assessment and Management of Adult Obesity
American Medical Association (AMA)
www.ama-assn.org/ama/pub/category/10931.html
Clinical tools for obesity management.
Free to use.

Obesity
Endotext.com
www.endotext.org/obesity/index.htm
> Academic review of health implications of obesity.
> Free to use.

"Evaluation and Treatment of Childhood Obesity"
American Family Physician, 1999
Rebecca Moran, MD,
www.aafp.org/afp/990215ap/861.html
> Nice review.
> Free to use.

Obesity in Pediatrics
eMedicine
www.emedicine.com/ped/topic1699.htm
> Academic review of childhood obesity.
> Free to use.

"The Clinical Picture of Metabolic Syndrome"
Postgraduate Medicine, 2004
Gregory C. Doelle, MD
www.postgradmed.com/issues/2004/07_04/doelle.htm
> Good clinical review of metabolic syndrome.
> Free to use.

Overweight Children and Adolescents
Maternal and Child Health Library
Georgetown University, Washington, DC
**www.mchlibrary.info/KnowledgePaths/
kp_overweight.html**
> Excellent resources.
> Free to use.

Overweight and Obesity
American Academy of Pediatrics (AAP)
www.aap.org/obesity
> Childhood obesity.
> Comprehensive academic review of the problems with overweight and obesity in childhood.
> Free to use.

Rudd Center for Food Policy and Obesity
Yale University—New Haven, Connecticut
www.yaleruddcenter.org
> Comprehensive obesity resource.
> Free to use.

Metabolic Syndrome
Medline Plus
National Library of Medicine (NLM)
www.nlm.nih.gov/medlineplus/metabolicsyndrome.html
> Extensive clinical resources.
> Free to use.

Obesity and the Metabolic Syndrome in Children and Adolescents
The New England Journal of Medicine (NEJM), 2004
Sonia Caprio, MD
http://content.nejm.org/cgi/content/abstract/350/23/2362
> Good clinical review of the Metabolic Syndrome. Registration, purchase, or subscription required.

Obstetrics and Gynecology (OB/GYN)/Women's Health ∽

Obstetrics Notebook
Family Practice Notebook
www.fpnotebook.com/OB.htm
> Family medicine resource on obstetrics.
> Free to use, but subscription option is available.

Contemporary OB/GYN
Advanstar Communications
www.contemporaryobgyn.net/obgyn/
> Journal covering OB/GYN, reproduction, oncology, and more.
> Subscription required, but online materials are free.

Contraception Online
Baylor College of Medicine—Houston, Texas
www.contraceptiononline.org
> Online contraceptive resource for clinicians, researchers, and educators.
> Free to use.

OBGYN.net
www.obgyn.net
> Extensive resource for women's health. Review "Medical Professionals" section and much more.
> Free to use.

ObGynLinx
www.mdlinx.com/obgynlinx/
> OB/GYN literature review. See "Resource Center."
> Free to use.

Journal of Obstetrics and Gynecology
Library of the National Medical Society
www.medical-library.org/j_obg.htm
> Journal of advances in OB/GYN.
> Registration required.

Women's Health
Journal Watch
http://womens-health.jwatch.org
> Literature review of women's health.
> Subscription required.

OB/GYN and Women's Health
Medscape
www.medscape.com/womenshealth
> Excellent clinical resource.
> Registration required.

Obstetrics and Gynecology
The American College of Obstetricians
and Gynecologists
Lippincott Williams & Wilkins
www.greenjournal.org
> Professional OB/GYN journal.
> Subscription required.

Maternal and Child Health Library
Georgetown University—Washington, DC
www.mchlibrary.info

Excellent educational resources. User must search the listed topics.

Free to use.

Women-Related Statements/Guidelines
American Heart Association (AHA)
www.americanheart.org/presenter.jhtml?identifier= 3020323

Collection of evidence-based clinical statements and guidelines for women. Check "Go Red for Women."

Free to use.

Obstetrics/Gynecology
eMedicine
www.emedicine.com/med/OBSTETRICSGYNECOLOGY .htm

Academic article collecton on Women's Health.

Free to use.

Oncology/Cancer ✑

National Cancer Institute (NCI)
National Institutes of Health (NIH)
http://www.cancer.gov

General cancer information resource. Comprehensive.
Free to use.

OncoLink
Abramsom Cancer Center of the University of Pennsylvania—Philadelphia, Pennsylvania
www.oncolink.com

Excellent, comprehensive academic resource covering all cancer topics.
Free to use.

Cancernetwork.com
www.cancernetwork.com

Cancer information resource.
Registration required.

Journal of Clinical Oncology
American Society of Clinical Oncology
http://jco.ascopubs.org

Academic journal covering clinical oncology.
Subscription required.

FDA Oncology Tools
www.fda.gov/cder/cancer
   Information related to cancer and approved cancer drug
treatments.
   Free to use.

World Oncology Network
www.worldoncology.net
   Expansive cancer resource for professionals.
   Free to use.

Oncology Collection
The New England Journal of Medicine (NEJM)
http://content.nejm.org/cgi/collection/oncology
   Collection of oncology articles.
   Register, purchase or subscribe.

Anti-cancer Drugs
Lippincott Williams & Wilkins
www.lww.com/product/?0959-4973
   Chemotherapy journal drug reviews.
   Subscription required.

Cancer
BioMed Central
www.biomedcentral.com/bmccancer
   Online oncology journal.
   Free to use.

Cancer Information Service
National Cancer Institute (NCI)
http://cis.nci.nih.gov
> National cancer information and education network.
> Free to use.

Cancer Literature in PubMed
National Cancer Institute (NCI)
www.cancer.gov/search/cancer_literature
> Search PubMed for cancer literature.
> Free to use.

Dose Calc Online
www.meds.com/DChome.html
> Oncology dosage calculations.
> Free to use.

Surveillance Epidemiology and End Results (SEER)
National Cancer Institute (NCI)
http://seer.cancer.gov
> Providing information on cancer statistics to help reduce the burden of cancer on the U.S. population.
> Free to use.

National Comprehensive Cancer Network
www.nccn.org
> Educational resources for professionals and patients.
> Free to use online.

Ophthalmology/Eye Disorders ✍

Archives of Ophthalmology
American Medical Association (AMA)
http://archopht.ama-assn.org
> Official AMA journal.
> Registration/subscription required.

Review of Ophthalmology
Jobson Publishing, LLC
www.revophth.com
> Professional ophthalmology journal.
> Subscription required.

Ophthalmology
eMedicine
www.emedicine.com/OPH
> Comprehensive academic ophthalmology resource.
> Free to use.

Ophthalmology
BioMed Central
www.biomedcentral.com/bmcophthalmol
> Online ophthalmology journal.
> Free to use.

Ophthalmology
American Academy of Ophthalmology (AAO)
www.ophsource.org/periodicals/ophtha
Official journal of the AAO.
Subscription required.

The Robert Bendheim Digital Atlas of Ophthalmology
The New York Eye and Ear Infirmary—New York, New York
www.nyee.edu/digital-atlas-of-ophthalmology.html
Digital eye atlas.
Free to use.

Eye Atlas of Ophthalmology
Oculisti Online
www.eyeatlas.com
Extensive collection of eye images.
Free to use.

The David G. Cogan Ophthalmic Pathology Collection
National Eye Institute (NEI)
National Institutes of Health (NIH)
http://cogancollection.nei.nih.gov
Extensive collection of eye disorders.
Free to use.

Ophthalmology Grand Rounds
EyeRounds.org
University of Iowa Health Care—Iowa City, Iowa
http://webeye.ophth.uiowa.edu/eyeforum
Excellent academic information reviewing eye disorders.
Free to use.

The Digest Eye
The University of Illinois Eye and Ear Infirmary Chicago, Illinois
www.agingeye.net

Review of cataracts, glaucoma, macular degeneration, diabetic retinopathy, and more.

Free to use.

Red Atlas
The Doheny Eye Institute
Keck School of Medicine
University of Southern California—Los Angeles, California
www.redatlas.org/main.htm

A visual review of eye disorders. Click "Quiz" to begin viewing images of the following: Anterior Segment, Glaucoma, Neuro-Ophthalmology, Oculoplastics, Pathology, Retina, and Uveitis.

Free to use.

Atlas of Ophthalmology
The International Council of Ophthalmology
www.atlasophthalmology.com

A public online database reviewing eye diseases. Multilanguage database in English, German, Spanish, Japanese, Russian, and Chinese.

Free to use.

Organa Donation ∾

The following sites are free resources on organ/tissue donation.

United Network for Organ Sharing (UNOS)
www.unos.org

Coalition on Donation—Donate Life
www.shareyourlife.org

Organ and Tissue Donation Initiative
www.organdonor.gov

Organ Donation
A Health Spotlight Special Report
PBS
www.pbs.org/newshour/health/organ-donation/
index.html

The Gift of a Lifetime
www.organtransplants.org

Organ Donation
Don't Let Myths Stand in Your Way

Mayo Clinic—Rochester, Minnesota
www.mayoclinic.com/health/organ-donation/FL00077

Living Organ Donor
www.livingorgandonor.org

Orthopedics/Bone Disorders ❧

Wheeless' Textbook of Orthopedics
Duke University Medical Center, Division of Orthopedic Surgery—Durham, North Carolina
Data Trace Internet Publishing Company
www.wheelessonline.com

> Comprehensive online orthopedic text.
>
> Free to use.

OrthoSupersite
www.orthosupersite.com

> Extensive academic information for orthopedics.
>
> Registration required.

American Journal of Orthopedics
Quadrant HealthCom Inc.
www.amjorthopedics.com

> Professional orthopedic journal.
>
> Subscription required.

Orthopedics Notebook
Family Practice Notebook
www.fpnotebook.com/ORT.htm

> General orthopedic reference for primary care.
>
> Free to use, but a subscription option is available.

Orthopaedics
Medscape
www.medscape.com/orthopaedics
> Extensive academic resource.
> Registration required.

Journal of Pediatric Orthopaedics
Lippincott Williams & Wilkins
www.pedorthopaedics.com
> Official journal of the European and North American Pediatric
> Orthopaedic Society.
> Subscription required.

Video Journal of Orthopaedics
Stanford University Libraries' Highwire Press
www.vjortho.com
> Online video orthopedic resource.
> Subscription/purchase required.

Orthopedic Surgery
eMedicine
www.emedicine.com/orthoped/index.shtml
> Academic article collection of orthopedic topics.
> Free to use.

Otolaryngology/Ears, Nose, and Throat ✍

Atlas of Head and Neck Pathology
The Ohio State University Medical Center—
Columbus, Ohio
Department of Otolaryngology—Head
and Neck Surgery
William H. Saunders, MD, and Paul Wakely Jr, MD
http://ent.osu.edu/7413.cfm

Ear, Nose, and Throat pathology atlas.

Free to use.

Otolaryngology and Facial Plastic Surgery
eMedicine
www.emedicine.com/ent/contents.htm

Extensive academic ENT resources.

Free to use.

Otolaryngology Core Curriculum Syllabus
Baylor College of Medicine—Houston, Texas
www.bcm.edu/oto/studs/toc.html

Academic teaching review of clinical ENT.

Free to use.

Archives of Otolaryngology—Head and Neck Surgery
American Medical Association (AMA)
http://archotol.ama-assn.org
    Academic ENT journal.
    Registration/subscription required.

Otolaryngology—Pediatrics
American Academy of Pediatrics Grand Rounds
http://aapgrandrounds.aappublications.org/cgi/
collection/otolaryngology
    Collection of pediatric ENT articles.
    Subscription required.

ENT Journal
Vendome Group, LLC
www.entjournal.com
    Online ENT journal.
    Subscription required.

Dr. Quinn's Online Textbook of Otolaryngology
ENT Grand Rounds
The University of Texas Medical Branch—
Galveston, Texas
www.utmb.edu/otoref/grnds/grndsindex.html
    Extensive collection of ENT grand rounds.
    Free to use.

Otolaryngology Notebook
Family Practice Notebook
www.fpnotebook.com/ENT.htm
    Primary care ENT review.
    Free to use, but a subscription option is available.

Current Opinion in Otolaryngology and Head and Neck Surgery
Lippincott Williams & Wilkins
www.lww.com/product/?1068-9508
Comprehensive ENT review.
Subscription required.

Ear, Nose, and Throat Disorders
BioMedCentral
www.biomedcentral.com/bmcearnosethroatdisord
Online, free access ENT journal.
Free to use.

Pain ✑

Cancer Pain Management in Children
Texas Children's Cancer Center—Houston, Texas
www.childcancerpain.org
> Professional site for pediatric pain.
> Free to use.

Pediatric Pain
Pediatric Pain Research Lab
Dalhousie University—Halifax, Nova Scotia, Canada
http://pediatric-pain.ca
> Pediatric pain management.
> Free to use.

Pain Management: Pediatric Pain Management
American Medical Association (AMA)
www.ama-cmeonline.com/pain_mgmt/module06
> Comprehensive and educational pediatric resources.
> CME online.

Pediatric Cancer Pain
National Comprehensive Cancer Network
www.nccn.org/professionals/physician_gls/PDF/
pediatric_pain.pdf
> Comprehensive pediatric pain guidelines.
> Free to use.

The Journal of Pain
Elsevier for the American Pain Society
www.us.elsevierhealth.com/product.jsp?
isbn=15265900
> Academic pain journal for The American Pain Society.
> Subscription required.

Pain Medicine
Blackwell Publishing
www.blackwellpublishing.com/journal.asp?
ref=1526=2375&site=1
> Official journal of the American Academy of Pain Medicine.
> Subscription required.

Pain Management
Amedeo—The Medical Literature Guide
www.amedeo.com
> Comprehensive literature review on pain management. Click on
> "Pain Management" in index.
> Registration required.

Therapeutic Injections for Pain Management
eMedicine
www.emedicine.com/neuro/topic514.htm
> Review of therapeutic injections for acute and chronic pain.
> Free to use.

Expert Guide to Pain Management
American College of Physicians (ACOP)
www.acponline.org/atpro/timssnet/catalog/books/
pain_management.htm?acp4037
> Book on pain management.
> Purchase required.

Pain Management Resource Center
American Academy of Physician Assistants
www.aapa.org/clinissues/pain/med-ed.html
> Review "Pain Management Resource Center."
> Free to use.

PainEDU.org
www.painedu.org
> Site for improving pain treatment through education.
> Free to use.

Pharmacologic Management of Pain
Medscape
www.medscape.com/resource/rxmgmtpain
> Extensive pain management resources.
> Registration required.

Advanced Approaches to Chronic Pain Management
Medscape
www.medscape.com/resource/painmgmt
> Clinical approach to intractable pain.
> Registration required.

Journal of Pain and Symptom Management Elsevier
www.elsevier.com/wps/find/journaldescription.cws_home/505775/description#description

Academic journal advancing pain symptom research, hospice, and palliative care.

Subscription required.

Parkinson's Disease ∽

Parkinson's Disease
Medscape
www.medscape.com/resource/parkinsons
> Good clinical and research information resource.
> Registration required.

Parkinson's Disease
Medline Plus
National Library of Medicine (NLM)
www.nlm.nih.gov/medlineplus/parkinsonsdisease.html
> Thorough listing of Parkinson references.
> Free to use.

Parkinson Disease
eMedicine
www.emedicine.com/NEURO/topic304.htm
> Clinical review of Parkinson's Disease and other related topics.
> Free to use.

"Parkinson's Disease: Diagnosis and Treatment"
American Family Physician, 2006
Shobha S. Rao, MD
www.aafp.org/afp/20061215/2046.html
> Clinical review of Parkinson's Disease evaluation and treatment.
> Free to use.

Parkinson's Disease Information Page
National Institute of Neurological Disorders and Stroke (NINDS)
National Institutes of Health (NIH)
www.ninds.nih.gov/disorders/parkinsons_disease/ parkinsons_disease.htm

> Good Parkinson's disease references. User must search.
> Free to use.

Parkinson's Disease
National Human Genome Research Institute
National Institutes of Health (NIH)
www.genome.gov/10001217

> General review of Parkinson's and heredity.
> Free to use.

Parkinson's Disease/Parkinsonism
Neurology
www.neurology.org/cgi/collection/parkinsons_disease_ parkinsonism#loopSniff

> Academic collection of articles on Parkinson's. Review "Related Collections."
> Subscription required.

The Michael J. Fox Foundation
for Parkinson's Research
www.michaeljfox.org

> Foundation focusing on a cure and research for Parkinson's. Review "Living with Parkinson's" and more.
> Free to use.

Pathology/Tissue Medicine ∽

WebPath
The Internet Pathology Laboratory for Medical Education
http://library.med.utah.edu/WebPath/webpath.html

Excellent pathology resource.

Free to use, but some purchases required.

PERLjam Pathology Images
Indiana University—Indianapolis, Indiana
http://erl.pathology.iupui.edu

Extensive selection of pathology materials.

Free to use.

PathConsult
Elsevier, Inc.
www.pathconsultddx.com

Extensive pathology resources for differential diagnosis.

Subscription required.

Case of the Month
Department of Pathology
University of Pittsburgh School of Medicine—
Pittsburgh, Pennsylvania
http://path.upmc.edu/casemonth.html

Extensive collections of anatomic and clinical pathology resources. Also review "Case Studies" for more pathology discussions.

Free to use.

Pathmax
Shawn E. Cowper, MD
www.pathmax.com
> Comprehensive pathology links, but user must search.
> Free to use.

Cytopathnet
www.cytopathnet.org/tiki-index.php
> Online resource for cytopathology.
> Free to use.

The Pathology Guy
www.pathguy.com
> Review the following links for resources: "Pathology Topics",
> "General Pathology", and "The Medical Teacher."
> Free to use.

The American Journal of Pathology
The American Society for Investigative Pathology
http://ajp.amjpathol.org
> Academic pathology journal.
> Subscription required.

Pathology Case Reviews
Lippincott Williams & Wilkins
www.pathologycasereviews.com
> Academic pathology journal.
> Subscription required.

Patient Rights/Advocacy ∽

Patient Rights
Medline Plus
National Library of Medicine (NLM)
www.nlm.nih.gov/medlineplus/patientrights.html

Thorough general reference for patient rights.

Free to use.

Medical Privacy
National Standards to Protect the Privacy
of Personal Health Information
U.S. Department of Health and Human Services
www.hhs.gov/ocr/hipaa

Comprehensive site on patient medical privacy and much more.

Free to use.

Communicating with Patients
American Hospital Association
www.aha.org/aha/issues/Communicating-With-Patients/index.html

Institutional review for improving patient communications.

Free to use.

Hospital Patient's Rights
IPRO
http://consumers.ipro.org/index/hospital-patients-rights
Extensive patient right's information primarily for New York, but other national resources are available.
Free to use.

Patient Rights
eMedicine
www.emedicinehealth.com/patient_rights/article_em.htm
Thorough general overview on patient rights.
Free to use.

The California Patient's Guide
www.calpatientguide.org
Excellent review for California patient rights. Review "En Español" for Spanish-speaking patients.
Free to use.

Patients' Rights in New York State
www.health.state.ny.us/professionals/patients/
patient_rights
Comprehensive review for New York patients. Multilingual sections available in Spanish, Italian, Russian, Greek, Chinese, Yiddish, and Creole.
Free to use.

Medicare Rights Center
www.medicarerights.org
Your information guide through the Medicare maze, covering patient rights.
Free to use.

Patient Advocacy Resources
Connecticut Consumer Health Information
University of Connecticut Health Center (UCHC)—
Farmington, Connecticut
http://library.uchc.edu/departm/hnet/advocacy.html

Comprehensive listing compiled by the UCHC library. User must search through links.

Free to use.

National Patient Advocate Foundation
www.npaf.org

A National Network for Healthcare Access. Review legislation and other current patient advocacy information.

Free to use.

Patient Safety ∽

Patient Safety
American College of Physicians (ACP)
www.acponline.org/ptsafety/?idx

Extensive resources.

Usage is mostly free, but membership in the ACP required.

National Patient Safety Foundation
www.npsf.org

Extensive resources.

Usage is mostly free, but some items require purchase.

Agency of Health Care Research and Quality
www.ahrq.gov/qual/errorsix.htm

Extensive professional resources on patient safety.

Free to use.

FDA Patient Safety News
U.S. Food and Drug Administration (FDA)
www.accessdata.fda.gov/scripts/cdrh/cfdocs/psn/
index.cfm

Reviews medical products, recalls, safety alerts, and patient
questions.

Free to use.

Patient Safety and Quality Healthcare
Lionheart Publishing, Inc.
www.psqh.com

Extensive resources on patient safety.

Free to use. Registration requires the user to sign-up for site entry.

Subscription requires a fee.

QuackWatch
www.quackwatch.org

A Web guide to quackery, health fraud, and intelligent decisions.

Web M&M
Morbidity & Mortality Rounds on the Web
Agency for Healthcare Research and Quality (AHRQ)
www.webmm.ahrq.gov

Case reviews and other resources on patient safety and health care quality.

Free to use.

Pediatrics/Childhood Medicine ∽

General Pediatrics
Donna M. D'Alessandro, MD
www.generalpediatrics.com
> Excellent pediatric resource. User must search links.
> Free to use.

Pediatrics
BioMed Central
www.biomedcentral.com/bmcpediatr
> Online pediatric journal.
> Free to use.

Child Neurology Home Page
Steven Leber, MD, PhD—University of Michigan
Kenneth Mack, MD, PhD—Mayo Clinic
www-personal.umich.edu/~leber/c-n
> Extensive pediatric clinical resources.
> Free to use.

National Immunization Program
Centers for Disease Control and Prevention (CDC)
www.cdc.gov/vaccines
> Extensive immunization resources, including information for adults.
> Free to use.

Immunization Action Coalition
www.immunize.org
> Extensive resources.
> Free to use.

Congenital Heart Information Network
http://tchin.org
> Good information on congenital heart disease.
> Free to use.

Pediatric Cardiology
Congenital Heart Defects
University of Kansas Medical Center—
Kansas City, Kansas
www.kumc.edu/gec/support/conghart.html
> Extensive resources. User must search through links.
> Free to use.

The Initiative for Pediatric Palliative Care
www.ippcweb.org
> Extensive educational materials.
> Free to use.

National Center on Birth Defects and
Developmental Disabilities
Centers for Disease Control and Prevention (CDC)
www.cdc.gov/ncbddd
> Extensive resources.
> Free to use.

National SIDS/Infant Death Resource Center
www.sidscenter.org
> Extensive resources.
> Free to use.

Online Pediatric Surgery Handbook
http://home.coqui.net/titolugo/handbook.htm
> Thorough pediatric surgical reference. See "Homepage."
> Free to use.

American Academy of Pediatrics (AAP)
www.aap.org
> Professional society dedicated to the health of all children.
> Subscription/membership required.

Pediatrics
American Academy of Pediatrics (AAP)
http://pediatrics.aappublications.org
> Official journal of the American Academy of Pediatrics.
> Subscription required.

Pediatrics in Review
American Academy of Pediatrics (AAP)
http://pedsinreview.aappublications.org
> Official journal of the American Academy of Pediatrics.
> Subscription required.

AAP Grand Rounds Subspecialty Collections
American Academy of Pediatrics (AAP)
http://aapgrandgrounds.aappublications.org/collections/
> Academic collection of pediatric subspecialty articles.
> Subscription required.

Pediatrics
eMedicine
www.emedicine.com/ped

Thorough pediatric subspecialty resources for medicine and surgery.

Free to use.

Child Neurology Society
www.childneurologysociety.org

Professional organization focusing on pediatric neurologic disease. Review "Practice Parameters" and "Physician Resources," especially "Practice Tools."

Usage is free, but memership required for certain sections.

This Week's ECG—Pediatrics
www.paedcard.com/files/archive.html

Collection of pediatric ECGs.

Free to use.

Girl Power
U.S. Department of Health and Human Services
www.girlpower.gov

A national public education campaign to help encourage and motivate 9 to 13 year-old girls to make the most of their lives.

Free to use.

GirlsHealth.gov
Office of Women's Health
U.S. Department of Health and Human Services
www.4girls.gov

Promoting healthy, positive behaviors in girls between the ages of 10 and 16.

Free to use.

PediNeuroLogic Exam
A Neurodevelopmental Approach
Paul D. Larsen, MD
Suzanne S. Stensaas, PhD
http://library.med.utah.edu/pedineurologicexam/html/ home_exam.html

Review neuroexam from newborn stage to two and a half years old.

Free to use.

PediatricEducation.org
Donna M. D'Alessandro, MD
Michael P. D'Alessandro, MD
www.pediatriceducation.org

An extensive pediatric virtual learning resource.

Free to use.

Pediatric Links
The American Academy of Pediatrics
New York Chapter
www.ny2aap.org/newyorkhome.htm#links.

Comprehensive collection of pediatric resources.

Free to use.

Pharmacology/Medication ✍

Thomson Micromedex
www.micromedex.com
    Comprehensive pharmacology database under "Solutions." Click on "Pharmacist." The pharmacology section includes information on drugs, toxicology, IV compatibility, interactions, and more.
    Subscription required.

PDR.net
www.pdr.net
    Online "Drug Information" with Drug Search, Interactions, Drug Alerts, and PDR Addenda.
    Registration required.

The Annals of Pharmacotherapy
Harvey Whitney Books Company
www.theannals.com
    Academic pharmacology journal.
    Subscription required.

Clinical Pharmacology
BioMed Central
www.biomedcentral.com/bmcclinpharmacol
    Open access pharmacology journal.
    Free to use.

Institute for Safe Medication Practices
www.ismp.org

Medication safety is the goal. Review professional materials on "Education and Awareness" and "Tools and Resources."

Some materials free to use; for others purchase required.

The Medical Letter
www.medletter.com

Excellent pharmacology review for prescription and nonprescription medications.

Subscription required.

MedWatch
The FDA Safety Information and Adverse Events Reporting Program
www.fda.gov/medwatch

An internet gateway for drug safety information.

Free to use.

Lexi-Comp
www.lexi.com

Extensive pharmacology database.

Purchase required.

Martindale's the Virtual Pharmacy, Pharmacology, and Toxicology Center
www.martindalecenter.com/Pharmacy.html

Extensive pharmacology resources, but user must search.

Free to use.

Malignant Hyperthermia Association of the United States (MHAUS)
www.mhaus.org
> Extensive clinical resources for MH.
> Although some materials are free, registration is required.

Neuroleptic Malignant Syndrome Information Service
www.nmsis.org
> Extensive resource on NMS.
> Usage is free, membership required.

ArizonaCERT-Drug-Induced Arrhythmias University of Arizona—Tucson, Arizona
www.qtdrugs.org
> Excellent resource on pro-arrhythmia drugs.
> Free to use.

Nephrology Pharmacy Associates
www.nephrologypharmacy.com
> Search "Publications" for educational materials on renal disease, Peritoneal Dialysis, drug interactions, dialysis of drugs, and more.
> Free to use.

Clinical Pharmacology Gold Standard
www.clinicalpharmacology.com
> Drug information databases, software and clinical information solutions.
> Purchase required.

Pediatric Pharmacotherapy
University of Virginia Children's Hospital—
Charlottesville, Virginia
www.healthsystem.virginia.edu/internet/pediatrics/
Academic selection of pediatric pharmacology topics. Click "Pharmacology Newsletter."
Free to use.

Cytochrome P450 Drug Interactions
Indiana University, Indianapolis, Indiana
http://medicine.iupui.edu/flockhart/table.htm
Spectacular and comprehensive.
Free to use.

RxMed
www.rxmed.com
Good general reference site. Review "Pharmceutical Information" and "Herbal & Dietary Supplements."
Free to use.

Drugs, Supplements, and Herbal Information
Medline Plus
National Library of Medicine (NLM)
www.nlm.nih.gov/medlineplus/druginformation.html
Search the comprehensive index.
Free to use.

Postpartum Depression (PPD) ∽

Postpartum Depression
eMedicine
www.emedicine.com/med/topic3408.htm

An academic review with related topics covering postpartum depression.

Free to use.

Postpartum Major Depression
C. Neill Epperson, MD
Yale University School of Medicine—New Haven, Connecticut
www.aafp.org/afp/990415ap/2247.html

A thorough clinical review.

Free to use.

Postpartum Depression
Medline Plus
National Library of Medicine (NLM)
www.nlm.nih.gov/medlineplus/postpartum depression.html

Great general resource.

Free to use.

"Postpartum Depression"
The New England Journal of Medicine, 2002
Katherine L. Wisner, MD, et al
http://content.nejm.org/cgi/content/extract/
347/3/194

> Thorough academic clinical review.
>
> Registration, purchase, or subscription required.

Postpartum Depression
University of Michigan Depression Center—
Ann Arbor, Michigan
www.med.umich.edu/depression/postpartum.htm

> Good general review, plus a "Women and Depression" section.
>
> Free to use.

Postpartum Depression
Maternal and Child Health Library
Georgetown University—Washington, DC
http://mchlibrary.info/KnowledgePaths/kp_
postpartum.html

> Excellent link resources, but user must search.
>
> Free to use.

Pregnancy Risk Assessment Monitoring System (PRAMS)
PRAMS and Postpartum Depression
Centers for Disease Control and Prevention (CDC)
www.cdc.gov/prams/PPD.htm

> Statistical factsheet on postpartum depression.
>
> Free to use.

Postpartum Depression
OBGYN.net
www.obgyn.net/femalepatient/default.asp?page=leopold

An excellent clinical review on a comprehensive women's health website.

Free to use.

Pregnancy and Lactation Drug Safety ℘

Drugs in Pregnancy and Breastfeeding
Perinatology.com
www.perinatology.com/exposures/druglist.htm

Excellent medication resources and other references.

Free to use, but other sites may require registration or a fee.

Drugs and Lactation Database (LactMed)
National Library of Medicine (NLM)
http://toxnet.nlm.nih.gov/cgi-bin/sis/htmlgen?LACT

Comprehensive drug and lactation resource.

Free to use.

ReproTox
www.reprotox.org

An information system on environmental hazards to human reproduction and development.

Subscription required.

National Toxicology Program (NTP)
NTP Center for the Evaluation of Risks to Human Reproduction
National Institutes of Health (NIH)
http://cerhr.niehs.nih.gov

Resource for the latest information about potentially hazardous effects of chemicals on human reproduction and development.

Free to use.

ReproRisk
Thomson/Micromedex
www.micromedex.com/products/reprorisk

Excellent databases to help evaluate human reproductive risks of drugs and chemical and physical/environmental agents.

Purchase required.

Breastfeeding Pharmacology
Thomas W. Hale, RPh, PhD
Texas Tech University Health Sciences Center— Amarillo, Texas
http://neonatal.ttuhsc.edu/lact

Thorough academic resource.

Free to use.

Drugs in Pregnancy and Lactation
A Reference Guide to Fetal and Neonatal Risk
Gerald G. Briggs, BPharm, et al
www.lww.com/product/?978-0-7817-5651-8

Expansive academic reference.

Purchase required.

Prescription Assistance Programs ✍

Partnership for Prescription Assistance
www.pparx.org/Intro.php

Extensive resources for prescription medication assistance for patients, caregivers, and professionals.

Usage is free, but application for medication assistance is required. Fee for medications may be necessary as determined by financial status.

Needy Meds
www.needymeds.com

Comprehensive resource for prescription medication assistance.

Usage is free, but application and fee for medications may be necessary.

CARxE
www.carxe.org

Provides and compares information about the Medicare approved drug plans as well as reviews the "Coverage Gap."

Free to use.

RxHope
www.rxhope.com
    An online patient assistance portal. Locate patient assistance programs by manufacturer, state and federal government, and pharmaceutical.
    Free to use.

Helping with Prescription Drug Costs
Social Security Online
www.ssa.gov/prescriptionhelp
    Resource for Medicare beneficiaries who may qualify for prescription assistance if they have limited income and resources.
    Free to use.

State Pharmaceutical Assistance Program
Medicare
www.medicare.gov/spap.asp
    Select a listed state for prescription assistance resources.
    Review the link on the "Coverage Gap."
    Free to use.

State Pharmaceutical Assistance Programs
National Conference of State Legislatures
www.ncsl.org/programs/health/drugaid.htm
    Comprehensive site covering legislation, assistance programs, and 2007 federal poverty guidelines.
    Free to use.

RxAssist
www.rxassist.org
    Comprehensive database for patient assistance programs on free and low-cost medications.
    Free to use.

TogetherRxAccess
www.togetherrxaccess.com

Resources for non-Medicare patients without prescription drug coverage who may apply for medication assistance.

Application and fee may be required.

Preventive Medicine/
Prevention ✐

Preventive Medicine
Family Practice Notebook
www.fpnotebook.com/PRE.htm
> Clinical resources for preventive medicine.
> Free to use, but a subscription option is available.

American Journal of Preventive Medicine
Elsevier
www.ajpm-online.net
> Professional journal for prevention research, teaching, practice, and policy.
> Subscription required.

Public Health and Prevention
Medscape
www.medscape.com/publichealth
> Excellent clinical resources.
> Registration required.

Preventing Chronic Disease
Centers for Disease Control and Prevention (CDC)
www.cdc.gov/pcd
> Comprehensive academic resource.
> Free to use.

Put Prevention into Practice
Agency for HealthCare Research and Quality (AHRQ)
www.ahrq.gov/clinic/ppipix.htm

Comprehensive reference for clinical preventive services.

Free to use.

Guide to Clinical Preventive Services
Agency for Healthcare Research & Quality (AHRQ)
www.ahrq.gov/clinic/gcpspu.htm

Excellent resources from the U.S. Preventive Services Task Force (USPSTF).

Free to use.

Preventive Medicine
MDLinx
**www.mdlinx.com/internalMDLinx/
news.cfm?subspec_id=484**

Review preventive medicine news.

Free to use but journal subscriptions required.

Public Health Links
American Public Health Association (APHA)
www.apha.org

Review "Resources" under "Programs and Resources" and more.

Free to use.

Public Health
BioMed Central
www.biomedcentral.com/bmcpublichealth

Online professional journal.

Free to use.

Office of Disease Prevention and Health Promotion
U.S. Department of Health and Human Services
http://odphp.osophs.dhhs.gov

Extensive resource for disease prevention and health promotion.

Free to use.

The National Center for HIV, STD, and TB Prevention
Centers for Disease Control and Prevention (CDC)
www.cdc.gov/nchstp/od/nchstp.html

Comprehensive prevention infectious disease resource.

Free to use.

Prostate Cancer ∾

**Prostate Cancer
Medline Plus
National Library of Medicine (NLM)**
www.nlm.nih.gov/medlineplus/prostatecancer.html
Good general resources for prostate cancer.
Free to use.

**Prostate Cancer
National Cancer Institute (NCI)
National Institutes of Health (NIH)**
www.cancer.gov/cancertopics/types/prostate
Excellent collection of resources on prostate cancer.
Free to use.

**Prostate Cancer
Online Mendelian Inheritance in Man (OMIM)
National Center for Biotechnology Information (NCBI)**
www.ncbi.nlm.nih.gov/entrez/dispomim.cgi?id=176807
Thorough review of the genetic factors for prostate cancer.
Free to use.

Prostate Cancer
Medscape
www.medscape.com/resource/prostate

Clinical reviews of prostate cancer, benign prostatic hypertrophy, and other prostate diseases.

Registration required.

"Prostate Cancer"
The New England Journal of Medicine (NEJM), 2003
William G. Nelson, MD, PhD, et al
http://content.nejm.org/cgi/content/short/349/4/366

Excellent clinical review with emphasis on genetic factors.

Registration, purchase, or subscription required.

Prostate Cancer: Metastatic and Advanced Disease
eMedicine
www.emedicine.com/med/topic3197.htm

Thorough review of prostate cancer and treatment options.

Free to use.

Prostate Cancer: Neoadjuvant Androgen Deprivation
eMedicine
www.emedicine.com/med/topic3396.htm

Academic review of hormonal manipulation in treating prostate cancer.

Free to use.

Guiding Prostate Cancer Treatment Choices
Postgraduate Medicine, 2005
Gregory T. Sweat, MD
www.postgradmed.com/issues/2005/04_05/sweat.htm

Nice review of prostate cancer treatment options.

Free to use.

Prostate Cancer
MD Anderson Cancer Center—Houston, Texas
www.mdanderson.org/diseases/prostate

Educational clinical resource for patients with prostate cancer.
Free to use.

Psychiatry/Mental Health ✑

Practice Guidelines
American Psychiatric Association (APA)
**www.psych.org/psych_pract/treatg/pg/
prac_guide.cfm**
>Clinical psychiatric guideline resource and more.
>Purchase may be required.

Psychiatry
BioMed Central
www.biomedcentral.com/bmcpsychiatry/
>Online psychiatry journal.
>Free to use.

Center for Effective Collaboration and Practice
http://cecp.air.org
>Extensive resource in children's mental health.
>Free to use.

National Institute of Mental Health (NIMH)
National Institutes of Health (NIH)
www.nimh.nih.gov/nimhhome/index.cfm
>Thorough general psychiatry resource. See "Clinical Trials."
>Free to use.

Psychiatry
Journal Watch
http://psychiatry.jwatch.org
Search the psychiatric literature.
Subscription required.

Psychiatry and Mental Health
Medscape
www.medscape.com/psychiatry
Excellent academic resource.
Registration required.

Disaster Mental Health Links
David Baldwin's Trauma Information Pages
www.trauma-pages.com/disaster.php
Multiple mental health resources for disaster victims. Extensive
listings for all diseases. User must search links.
Free to use.

Psychiatry 24×7
www.psychiatry24×7.com
Extensive resources for psychiatry, including disease information,
medline, educational tools, and drug interactions.
Registration required for professional access.

Psychiatry
eMedicine
www.emedicine.com/med/PSYCHIATRY.htm
Academic collection of psychiatry topics.
Free to use.

Psychiatry Notebook
Family Practice Notebook
www.fpnotebook.com/PSY.htm

Extensive psychiatry resources.

Free to use.

Publishers (Medical) ∽

Lippincott Williams & Wilkins
www.lww.com

McGraw-Hill
http://www.mhprofessional.com/category/?cat=116

Elsevier
(Saunders-Mosby-Churchill Livingstone-
Butterworth-Heinemann)
http://us.elsevierhealth.com

Humana Press
www.humanapress.com

BMJ Publishing Group
www.group.bmj.com

MedBioWorld
www.sciencekomm.at/publish.html
  Extensive listing of medical publishers.

Thieme
www.thieme.com

MacMillan
www.macmillan.com

Karger
www.karger.com

Oxford University Press
www.oup.co.uk

Slack, Inc.
www.slackinc.com

John Wiley & Sons, Inc.
www.wiley.com/WileyCDA/

BC Decker
www.bcdecker.com

Annual Reviews
www.annualreviews.org

Springer
www.springer.com

Blackwell
www.blackwellpublishing.com

Cambridge University Press
www.cambridge.org:80/uk/default.asp

The National Academies Press
www.nap.edu

Pulmonary/Respiratory Disease

Pulmonary
eMedicine
www.emedicine.com/med/PULMONOLOGY.htm
> Academic clinical article resource for lung diseases.
> Free to use.

The Drug-Induced Lung Diseases
Pneumotox Online
www.pneumotox.com
> Comprehensive listing of drugs that affect the lung, along with their clinical and radiographic patterns. Download program.
> Free to use.

The Global Initiative for Asthma (GINA)
www.ginasthma.org
> Resources for evidence-based guidelines for asthma management and more.
> Free downloads, but purchase required for print materials.

Practical Guide for the Diagnosis and Management of Asthma
National Heart, Lung, and Blood Institute (NHLBI)
National Institutes of Health (NIH)
www.nhlbi.nih.gov/health/prof/lung/asthma/practgde.htm
> Asthma clinical practice guidelines.
> Free download, but print copy requires purchase.

Pulmonary Function Testing
eMedicine
www.emedicine.com/med/topic2972.htm
Academic review.
Free to use.

Pulmonary Hypertension Association
www.phassociation.org/Medical
Thorough professional resources.
Free to use.

Asbestosis
eMedicine
www.emedicine.com/med/topic171.htm
Academic review.
Free to use.

Management of COPD: An Update
American Academy of Family Physicians
www.aafp.org/online/en/home/cme/selfstudy/videocme/
copdmanagement.html
Academic review with CME online.
Registration/subscription required.

Pulmonary Embolism
eMedicine
www.emedicine.com/med/topic1958.htm
Academic review.
Free to use.

Pleural Effusion
eMedicine
www.emedicine.com/emerg/topic462.htm
   Academic review.
   Free to use.

The Intricacies of Pneumothorax
Postgraduate Medicine Online
www.postgradmed.com/issues/2005/12_05/dincer.htm
   Good clinical review.
   Free to use.

Severe Acute Respiratory Syndrome (SARS)
Centers for Disease Control and Prevention (CDC)
www.cdc.gov/ncidod/sars
   Excellent CDC review.
   Free to use.

Lung Diseases
Medline Plus
National Library of Medicine (NLM)
www.nlm.nih.gov/medlineplus/lungdiseases.html
   Thorough collection of resources.
   Free to use.

American Journal of Respiratory and Critical Care Medicine
American Thoracic Society (ATS)
http://ajrccm.atsjournals.org
   Official journal of the American Thoracic Society.
   Subscription required.

Pulmonary Medicine
BioMed Central
www.biomedcentral.com/bmcpulmmed

Online pulmonary medicine journal.

Free to use.

Francis J. Curry—National Tuberculosis Center
University of California—San Francisco, California
www.nationaltbcenter.edu

Clinical tuberculosis (TB) reviews.

Download or purchase required.

Global Tuberculosis Institute
New Jersey Medical School, Newark, New Jersey
www.umdnj.edu/globaltb/home.htm

Extensive TB resources.

Free to use and/or purchases required.

National Jewish Medical and Research Center
Denver, Colorado
www.nationaljewish.org

Official site of the global leader in treating lung diseases.

Free to use.

Pulmonary
Family Practice Notebook
www.fpnotebook.com/LUN.htm

Good primary care review.

Free to use, but a subscription option is available.

American College of Chest Physicians
www.chestnet.org
> Extensive professional resources.
> Membership required but some materials free or for purchase.

Avian Influenza (Bird Flu)
Centers for Disease Control and Prevention (CDC)
www.cdc.gov/flu/avian/
> Excellent educational resource.
> Free to use.

Respiratory Research
BioMedCentral
http://respiratory-research.com
> Online respiratory research journal.
> Free to use.

Sleep Home Pages
www.sleephomepages.org
> Comprehensive sleep resource. User must search links.
> Free to use.

Sleep Medicine
www.elsevier.com
> Academic sleep journal. Search "Sleep Medicine."
> Subscription required.

The Sleep Medicine Homepage
www.users.cloud9.net/~thorpy
> Extensive sleep resources. Users must review links.
> Free to use.

The New York State Smoker's Quitsite
www.nysmokefree.com/newweb/default.aspx
Smoking cessation.
Free to use.

QuitNet
www.quitnet.com
Smoking cessation site in cooperation with Boston University
School of Public Health.
Free to use.

Smoking Cessation
Medline Plus
National Library of Medicine (NLM)
www.nlm.nih.gov/medlineplus/smokingcessation.html
Comprehensive resources for smoking cessation.
Free to use.

Smokefree.gov
www.smokefree.gov
Excellent resource for smoking cessation.
Free to use.

Pulmonary Rehabilitation
Joint ACCP/AACVPR Evidence-Based Clinical Practice
Guidelines Chest, 2007
www.chestjournal.org/cgi/content/full/131/5_suppl/45
Academic review of pulmonary rehabilitation.
Free to use.

Radiology ✑

PediatricRadiology.com: A Pediatric Radiology Digital Library
Michael P. D'Alessandro, MD
www.pediatricradiology.com

Extensive pediatric radiology and pediatric imaging digital library.

Free to use.

Radiology Rounds
MDChoice
www.mdchoice.com/xray/xrx.asp

Collection of plain radiographs and CT scans by diagnosis.

Free to use.

Medical Imaging
BioMed Central
www.biomedcentral.com/bmcmedimaging

Online radiology journal.

Free to use.

CTisus
www.CTisus.com

Interesting CT/PET educational site.

Free to use and purchases required.

Iowa Neuroradiology Library
University of Iowa Hospitals and Clinics—Iowa City, Iowa
www.uiowa.edu/~c064s01/
> Extensive neuroradiology teaching files.
> Free to use.

The Whole Brain Atlas
Harvard Medical School—Boston, Massachusetts
www.med.harvard.edu/AANLIB/home.html
> Extensive neuroradiology teaching files.
> Free to use.

MedPix
Medical Image Database
http://rad.usuhs.edu/medpix/index.html
> Extensive radiology teaching files and imaging atlas.
> Free to use.

Nuclear Medicine Teaching File
Mallinckrodt Teaching File
Washington University—St. Louis, Missouri
http://gamma.wustl.edu/home.html
> Extensive nuclear medicine teaching file.
> Free to use.

Online Teaching Materials
University of Washington—Seattle, Washington
Department of Radiology
www.rad.washington.edu/teachingfiles.html
> Diverse selection of teaching files, including mammography.
> Free to use.

Radiology Education
Michael P. D'Alessandro, MD
www.radiologyeducation.com

A digital library of extensive radiology education resources. User must search the links.

Free to use.

Radiology
eMedicine
www.emedicine.com/radio/index.shtml

Clinical radiology topic review.

Free to use.

Chest X-ray Atlas
Loyola University Medical Center—Chicago, Illinois
A. J. Chandrasekhar, MD
www.meddean.luc.edu/lumen/meded/medicine/
pulmonar/cxr/atlas/cxratlas_f.htm

Extensive chest radiograph collection.

Free to use.

EuroRad
European Association of Radiology E-Learning Initiative
www.eurorad.org

Excellent clinical radiology resource.

Registration required.

X-Rays
Medline Plus
National Library of Medicine (NLM)
www.nlm.nih.gov/medlineplus/xrays.html

General radiology resource.

Free to use.

BrighamRAD
Brigham and Women's Hospital—Boston, Massachusetts
http://brighamrad.harvard.edu/index.html

Very educational RadPath Collection and BrighamRAD Teaching File.

Free to use.

Rare Diseases ✌

National Organization of Rare Disorders (NORD)
www.rarediseases.org

Extensive database for rare diseases.

Some materials are free, but others may require subscription or a fee.

Office of Rare Diseases
National Institutes of Health (NIH)
http://rarediseases.info.nih.gov

Excellent resource for clinical information on rare diseases.

Free to use.

Rare Diseases
Health on the Net Foundation (HON)
www.hon.ch/HONselect/RareDiseases

Extensive listing of diseases and more information.

Free to use.

Orphanet
Paris, France
www.orpha.net

Database dedicated to information on rare diseases and orphan drugs.

Free to use.

Genetic and Rare Conditons Site
University of Kansas Medical Center—
Kansas City, Kansas
www.kumc.edu/gec/support

Extensive disease listing, but users must search the links.

Free to use.

Rheumatology/Arthritis and Musculoskeletal Disorders ∽

Rheumatology
eMedicine
www.emedicine.com/med/Rheumatology.htm
> Extensive contents for rheumatology disorders.
> Free to use.

Rheumatology Notebook
Family Practice Notebook
www.fpnotebook.com/RHE.htm
> Extensive contents for rheumatology disorders in primary care.
> Free to use, but subscription option is available.

Rheumatology
Medscape
www.medscape.com/rheumatology
> Excellent clinical resources.
> Registration required.

National Institute of Arthritis and Musculoskeletal and Skin Diseases (NIAMS)
National Institutes of Health (NIH)
www.niams.nih.gov

General resource for arthritis, musculoskeletal, and skin diseases.

Free to use.

Rheumatology Clinical Guidelines
American College of Rheumatology
www.rheumatology.org/publications/index.asp

Academic clinical and research resource.

Free to use, but membership required.

Rheumatology Collection
British Medical Journal (BMJ)
http://bmj.com/cgi/collection/
rheumatology:other

Collection of rheumatology articles.

Subscription required.

Rheumatic Disease Collections
The New England Journal of Medicine (NEJM)
http://content.nejm.org/cgi/collection/
rheumatic_disease

Collection of rheumatology articles.

Registration, purchase, or subscription required.

Musculoskeletal Disorders
BioMed Central
www.biomedcentral.com/bmcmusculoskeletdisord/

Online journal for musculoskeletal disease.

Free to use.

Arthritis & Rheumatism
American College of Rheumatology
John Wiley & Sons, Inc.
www3.interscience.wiley.com/cgi-bin/jhome/76509746
Academic rheumatology journal.
Subscription required.

Arthritis
Medline Plus
National Library of Medicine (NLM)
www.nlm.nih.gov/medlineplus/arthritis.html
General arthritis resource.
Free to use.

Spinal Cord Injury (SCI) ∽

Spinal Cord Information Page
National Institute of Neurological Disorders
and Stroke (NINDS)
www.ninds.nih.gov/disorders/sci/sci.htm
    Good general resource.
    Free to use.

Spinal Cord Injuries
Medline Plus
National Library of Medicine (NLM)
www.nlm.nih.gov/medlineplus/spinalcordinjuries.html
    Extensive reference site.
    Free to use.

The Christopher and Dana Reeve Paralysis
Resource Center
www.paralysis.org
    Comprehensive spinal cord injury resource.
    Free to use.

Spinal Cord Injury Information Network
University of Alabama—Birmingham, Alabama
www.spinalcord.uab.edu
    Excellent resource. Review "SCI Topics."
    Free to use.

Spinal Cord Trauma and Related Disorders
eMedicine
www.emedicine.com/neuro/topic711.htm
Thorough clinical review of spinal cord injury and related disorders.
Free to use.

Spinal Cord Injury
eMedicine
www.emedicine.com/pmr/SPINAL_CORD_INJURY.htm
Academic clinical review of spinal cord injury.
Free to use.

Northwest Regional Spinal Cord
Injury System (NWRSCIS)
University of Washington—Seattle, Washington
http://sci.washington.edu/info/newsletters/index.asp
Review "SCI Update Newsletter," plus other resources.
Free to use.

Spinal Cord Injury Clinical Trials
National Institutes of Health (NIH)
www.clinicaltrials.gov/search/term=spinal+cord+Injury
Listing of SCI trials.
Free to use.

Spinal Cord Injury: Emerging Concepts, 2005
National Institute of Neurological Disorders
and Stroke (NINDS)
**www.ninds.nih.gov/news_and_events/proceedings/
sci_report.htm**
Extensive review of SCI.
Free to use.

Spinal Cord Injury: Progress, Promise and Priorities, 2005
The National Academies Press
http://www.nap.edu/catalog.php?record_id=11253

Comprehensive online review of SCI.

Free to use online or purchase required.

RehabTeamSite
PoinTIS
University of Miami School of Medicine— Miami, Florida
http://calder.med.miami.edu/pointis

Excellent resource for spinal cord injury and traumatic brain injury.

Free to use.

International Ventilator Users Network (IVUN)
www.ventusers.org

World's premier resource linking to experts in home mechanical ventilation.

Fees may be required for certain content.

Sports Medicine ✍

Medicine and Science in Sport and Exercise
Lippincott Williams & Wilkins
www.ms-se.com
> Official journal of the American College of Sports Medicine.
> Subscription required.

The American Journal of Sports Medicine
The American Orthopaedic Society for Sports Medicine
http://ajs.sagepub.com
> Professional journal.
> Subscription required.

Nicholas Institute of Sports Medicine and Athletic Trauma
Lenox Hill Hospital—New York, New York
www.nismat.org
> Good sports medicine resource with pictoral/video guide to
> exercise and rehabilitation protocols.
> Free to use.

Ackland Sports Medicine
New England Baptist Hospital—Boston, Massachusetts
www.sportismedicine.com
> General resource including adults, children, and elderly.
> Free to use.

Sports Medicine
eMedicine
www.emedicine.com/sports
> Academic collection on sports medicine.
> Free to use.

Clinical Journal of Sports Medicine
Lippincott Williams & Wilkins
www.cjsportmed.com
> Clinical journal for sports medicine.
> Subscription required.

British Journal of Sports Medicine
http://bjsm.bmj.com
> Archive collection of online issues.
> Subscription required.

The Stretching Handbook
www.thestretchinghandbook.com
> Stretching exercise review.
> Free to use online.

Sports Medicine and Fitness
American Academy of Pediatrics (AAP)
www.aap.org/sections/sportsmedicine
> Comprehensive sports medicine resource for children.
> Free to use.

American Academy of Orthopaedic Surgeons
http://orthoinfo.aaos.org

Review the Patient Education Library—Sports/Exercise, for sports resources plus more.

Free to use.

Statistics (Medical) ✑

British Medical Journal: Statistics Notes
www.tufts.edu/~gdallal/bmj.htm
Exclusive collection of the finest series of short articles on medical statistics.
Free to use.

Medical Statistics at a Glance
Blackwell Publishing
www.medstatsaag.com
Review of medical statistics.
Purchase required.

An Introduction to Medical Statistics
Martin Bland
www-users.york.ac.uk/~mb55/intro/introcon.htm
Review of medical statistics.
Purchase required.

Essential Medical Statistics
Blackwell Publishing
www.blackwellpublishing.com/essentialmedstats
Academic medical statistics book.
Purchase required.

Biostatistics for the Clinician
University of Texas
Houston Health Science Center
www.uth.tmc.edu/uth_orgs/educ_dev/oser/osertoc.htm
Online biostatistics instruction.
Free to use.

Medical Research Methodology
BioMed Central
www.biomedcentral.com/bmcmedresmethodol
Online journal reviewing methodological approaches to health care research.
Free to use.

Statistics
The New England Journal of Medicine (NEJM)
http://content.nejm.org/cgi/collection/statistics
Academic collection of medical statistics.
Registration, purchase, or subscription required.

Stem Cells ✑

Stem Cell Information
National Institutes of Health (NIH)
http://stemcells.nih.gov
> Reference on the federal stem cell research issues.
> Free to use.

Stem Cells and Stem Cell Transplantation
MedLine Plus
National Institutes of Health (NIH)
www.nlm.nih.gov/medlineplus/stemcells.html
> Good general resource.
> Free to use.

SCDb: The Stem Cell Database
Princeton University/University of Pennsylvania
http://stemcell.princeton.edu
> Database of hematopoietic stem cell system.
> Free to use.

Stem Cell Research
PBS Online
MacNeil/Lehrer Productions
www.pbs.org/newshour/health/stemcells.html
> A health spotlight special report on stem cells.
> Free to use.

"The Stem Cell Debate"
Time, Inc., 2001
www.time.com/time/2001/stemcells
> Excellent discussion from 2001 on stem cell research.
> Free to use.

"The Politics and Promise of Stem Cell Research"
The New England Journal of Medicine (*NEJM*), 2006
Robert S. Schwartz, MD
http://content.nejm.org/cgi/content/full/355/12/1189
> Editorial overview on the current politics of stem cell research.
> Free to use.

Stem Cell
Institute for Regeneration Medicine
University of California—San Francisco, California
http://irm.ucsf.edu
> Academic site covering stem cell research.
> Free to use.

Embryonic Stem Cells
University of Wisconsin—Madison, Wisconsin
www.news.wisc.edu/packages/stemcells
> General resource site for stem cells.
> Free to use.

Stem Cells
AlphaMedPress
http://stemcells.alphamedpress.org
> Academic journal covering cell differentiation and proliferation.
> Subscription required.

Stem Cell Research
Amedeo
www.amedeo.com/medicine/stc.htm
> Search the medical literature guide for stem cell research.
> Free to use.

International Society for Stem Cell Research
www.isscr.org
> Professional society for stem cell research. Review "Stem Cell
> Science" for extensive resources and more.
> Free to use, but may require registration.

American Association for the Advancement
of Sciences (AAAS)
www.aaas.org
> Professional society and publisher of the journal *Science*.
> Search "stem cells" for resources.
> Free to use, but one may subscribe.

Monitoring Stem Cell Research
The President's Council on Bioethics
January 2004
www.bioethics.gov/reports/stemcell
> Comprehensive review on the bioethics of stem cell research.
> Free to use.

EuroStemCell
European Consortium for Stem Cell Research
www.eurostemcell.org
> A virtual European stem cell center.
> Free to use.

State Embryonic and Fetal Research Laws
National Conference of State Legislatures
www.ncsl.org/programs/health/Genetics/embfet.htm
> Extensive review of state statutes on embryonic and fetal re-
> search.
> Free to use.

Stem Cells at the National Academies
The National Academies
http://dels.nas.edu/bls/stemcells
> Scientific publications reviewing stem cell research.
> Free to use.

Stem Cell Research News
www.medicalnewstoday.com/sections/stem_cell/
> Scientific news releases on stem cell research.
> Free to use.

"Isolation of Amniotic Stem Cell Lines with Potential for Therapy"
Nature Biotechnology, 1/2007
Anthony Atala, et al
www.nature.com/nbt/journal/v25/n1/abs/nbt1274.html
> Review new findings on amniotic fluid-derived stem (AFS) cells.
> Subscription required.

Stem Cell Research and Therapy
Medscape
www.medscape.com/resource/stem-cell-research
Overview of stem cell applications.
Registration required.

Stress Management ✍

Critical Incident Stress Management
eMedicine
www.emedicine.com/emerg/topic826.htm
  Clinical review of stress and stress management.
  Free to use.

Stress Management Workshop Online
Georgia Southern University—Statesboro, Georgia
http://students.georgiasouthern.edu/counseling/
workshop/stress/stress01.html
  Online review of stress and stress management.
  Free to use.

Stress
Medline Plus
National Institutes of Health (NIH)
www.nlm.nih.gov/medlineplus/stress.html
  Thorough general overview of stress.
  Free to use.

Stress Center
Relaxation Techniques and Exercise
Mayo Clinic—Rochester, Minnesota
www.mayoclinic.com/health/stress/SR00026
  Review "Articles" and "Tools."
  Free to use.

Stress Management
About.com
http://mentalhealth.about.com/od/stress/
stress_management.htm

Indepth general review articles and resources covering stress and stress management. User must search links.

Free to use.

Stress
Aetna InteliHealth
Harvard Medical School—Boston, Massachusetts
www.intellihealth.com

Click "Stress" under "Diseases & Conditions." Review "Stress-Management Techniques" and more.

Free to use.

The Relaxation Response
Dr. Herbert Benson
www.vcn.bc.ca/rmdcmha/stressa.html

Excellent review of relaxation techniques—Relaxation Response, Muscle Relaxation, Deep Breathing, Visualization, Meditation, and Nature.

Free to use.

International Journal of Stress Management
American Psychology Association (APA)
www.apa.org/journals/str

Professional journal reviewing stress management.

Subscription required.

Tips for Managing Your Stress in College
University of Pittsburgh Student Health Services
**www.pitt.edu/~studhlth/studenthealthed_wbpage/
index.html**

Useful suggestions for stress management in college. Click "Stress Management" and then "Tips."

Free to use.

Stress Management
Academic Skills Center
Dartmouth College—Hanover, New Hampshire
www.dartmouth.edu/~acskills/videos/video_sm.html

Excellent video for college students covering stress and stress management.

Free to use.

Authentic Happiness
University of Pennsylvania—Philadephia, Pennsylvania
www.authentichappiness.sas.upenn.edu

A new branch of psychology that focuses on the empirical study of positive emotions, strength-based character, and healthy institutions.

Free to use.

Humor Matters
Steven M. Sultanoff, PhD
www.humormatters.com

Extensive and interesting site on humor. Users must search.

Free to use.

Association for Applied and Therapeutic Humor
www.aath.org

An international community of professionals who incorporate humor into their daily lives. Review "Humor Resources" and more.

Free to use.

Comprehensive Acute Traumatic Stress Management
The American Academy of Experts in Traumatic Stress
www.atsm.org

Collection of practical tools for addressing the wide spectrum of traumatic experiences.

Free online, but fee required for print edition.

Surgery ✑

Archives of Surgery
American Medical Association (AMA)
http://archsurg.ama-assn.org
> Professional surgery journal.
>
> Register, purchase, or subscribe.

Annals of Surgery
Lippincott Williams & Wilkins
www.annalsofsurgery.com
> The world's most highly referenced academic surgical journal.
>
> Subscription required.

Surgery
Mosby, Inc.
www.sciencedirect.com/science/journal/00396060
> Professional surgery journal.
>
> Subscription required.

Surgery
BioMed Central
www.biomedcentral.com/bmcsurg/
> Online surgery journal.
>
> Free to use.

Surgery Textbook
eMedicine
www.emedicine.com/specialties.htm
   Academic review including General Surgery, Neurosurgery, OB/GYN, Perioperative, Thoracic, Transplantation, Trauma, Urology, Vascular, and more. Search "Surgery."
   Free to use.

SurgeryLinx
www.mdlinx.com/surgerylinx
   Professional site for news and journal article reviews covering surgery.
   Free to use.

General Surgery
Medscape
www.medscape.com/generalsurgery
   General surgery clinical information.
   Registration required.

Vesalius
www.vesalius.com
   The Clinical Folios are a diverse collection of graphical educational narratives on surgical anatomy and procedures designed for online study and reference.
   Subscription required.

Anesthesiology and Surgery Center
Martindale's The "Virtual" Medical Center
www.martindalecenter.com/MedicalSurgery.html
   Collection of internet resources. User must search links.
   Free to use.

Pediatric Surgery
eMedicine

   a) www.emedicinecom/ped/GENERAL_SURGERY
      .htm
   b) www.emedicine/ped/CARDIOTHORACIC_SUR-
      GERY.thm
   c) www.emedicine.com/ped/VASCULAR_SURGERY
      .htm

   Academic collection of pediatric surgery articles.

   Free to use.

ACS Surgery: Principles and Practice
American College of Surgeons

www.acssurgery.com

   Comprehensive online surgical review.

   Subscription required.

Teratology/Causes of Abnormal Fetal Development ∽

The Visible Embryo
National Institutes of Child Health and
Human Development
www.visembryo.com
A comprehensive educational resource of human development.
Free to use.

Teratogen Information Systems (TERIS)
University of Washington—Seattle, Washington
http://depts.washington.edu/~terisweb/teris
Database for assessing the risk of possible teratogenic exposures
in pregnant women including Shepard's Catalog of Teratogenic
Agents.
Subscription required.

Teratology and Drug Use During Pregnancy
eMedicine
www.emedicine.com/med/topic3242.htm
Academic review of teratology and medication use during
pregnancy.
Free to use.

Organization of Teratology Information Specialists (OTIS)
http://otispregnancy.org
Great general resource site.
Free to use.

International Birth Defects Information Systems (IBIS)
www.ibis-birthdefects.org
Extensive clinical resources.
Free to use.

Human Embryology and Teratology, 3rd edition
Ronan R. O'Rahilly and Fabiola Müller
John Wiley & Sons, Inc.
www.wiley.com/WileyCDA/WileyTitle/productCd-0471382256.html
Exceptional medical reference.
Purchase required.

Toxicology/Toxins ✑

Toxnet
Toxicology Data Network
National Library of Medicine (NLM)
http://toxnet.nlm.nih.gov

Databases on toxicology, hazardous chemicals, environmental health, and toxic releases. Comprehensive.

Free to use.

Therapeutic Drug Monitoring
Lippincott Williams & Wilkins
www.drug-monitoring.com

Journal covering Clinical Pharmacology, Pathology, Toxicology, and Analytical Chemistry.

Subscription required.

Poisons Information Monographs
Canadian Centre for Occupational Health and Safety
www.inchem.org/pages/pims.html

Extensive information, covering Poisonous Plants, Poisonous Animals, Pharmaceuticals, Fungi, and Chemicals.

Free to use.

Medical Management Guidelines for Acute Chemical Exposures
Agency for Toxic Substances and Disease Registry
www.atsdr.cdc.gov/MHMI/mmg.html

Database for emergency healthcare professionals who manage acute chemical exposures.

Free to use.

The Natural Toxins Research Center
Texas A & M University—Kingsville, Texas
http://ntrc.tamuk.edu

Database on snake venoms.

Free to use.

Snakebite Protocols
University of California—San Diego, California
http://drdavidson.ucsd.edu/Portals/0/index.htm

Extensive resources on snakebites.

Free to use.

NBC Links
www.nbc-links.com

Extensive resources for nuclear, biologic, and chemical materials. Users must search links.

Free to use.

Chemical Warfare Agents
www.opcw.org/resp/html/cwagents.html

Detailed review of nerve agents, mustard agents, hydrogen cyanide, arsines, psychotomimetic agents, toxins, and more.

Free to use.

Mushroom Toxicity
eMedicine
www.emedicine.com/emerg/topic874.htm
Review of mushroom toxicity.
Free to use.

Diagnosis and Management of Foodborne Illnesses
Morbidity and Mortality Weekly Report (MMWR), 2001
Centers for Disease Control and Prevention (CDC)
www.cdc.gov/mmwr/preview/mmwrhtml/rr5002a1.htm
Foodborne illness review.
Free to use.

Recognition and Management of Pesticide Poisoning
U.S. Environmental Protection Agency (EPA)
www.epa.gov/pesticides/index.htm
Extensive resources covering pesticides.
Free to use.

Withdrawal Syndromes
eMedicine
www.emedicine.com/emerg/topic643.htm
Review of clinical withdrawal syndromes.
Free to use.

Clinical Toxinology Resources
Women's and Children's Hospital
Adelaide, Australia
www.toxinology.com
Extensive resource on first aid, snakes, spiders/scorpions, marine life, and plants.
Subscription required.

Toxicology
eMedicine
www.emedicine.com/emerg/TOXICOLOGY.htm
Extensive clinical article collection on poisons.
Free to use.

Streetdrugs.org
www.streetdrugs.org
Interesting site covering street drugs.
Free to use. Some content requires purchase.

National Institute on Drug Abuse (NIDA)
National Institues of Health (NIH)
www.nida.nih.gov/NIDAHome.html
Excellent resource on drugs and abuse.
Free to use.

Transplantation ∽

Transplant Patholog y Internet Services
University of Pittsburgh—Pittsburgh, Pennsylvania
http://tpis.upmc.edu
> Extensive transplant pathology resource.
> Free to use.

Transplantation
Medscape
www.medscape.com/transplantation
> Thorough professional transplantation resource.
> Registration required.

Transplantation
eMedicine
www.emedicine.com/med/TRANSPLANTATION.htm
> Extensive resource on all aspects of transplantation.
> Free to use.

Transplantation
Lippincott Williams & Wilkins
www.transplantjournal.com
> The official journal of the Transplantation Society.
> Subscription required.

Current Opinion in Organ Transplantation
Lippincott Williams & Wilkins
www.co-transplantation.com

Journal dedicated to selected topics in transplantation.
Subscription required.

Trauma ✑

Trauma.org
www.trauma.org
   Providing global education, information, and communication
resources for professionals in trauma and critical care.
   Free to use, but registration required for certain access.

The Eastern Association for the Surgery of Trauma
www.east.org
   Trauma practice guidelines. Adobe Acrobat required.
   Free to use.

Brain Trauma Foundation
www.braintrauma.org
   Guideline education for traumatic brain injury (TBI).
   Free to use, but some purchases required.

Liverpool Trauma Website
University of New South Wales—Sydney, Australia
Liverpool Hospital—Trauma Department
www.swsahs.nsw.gov.au/livtrauma/
   Extensive trauma education resource.
   Registration required.

The Journal of Trauma Injury, Infection, and Critical Care
Lippincott Williams & Wilkins
www.jtrauma.com
Professional trauma journal.
Subscription required.

Mass Casualty Event Preparedness and Response
Centers for Disease Control and Prevention (CDC)
www.bt.cdc.gov/masscasualties/
CDC site for mass trauma emergency preparedness and response.
Free to use.

Helping Young Children Cope with Trauma
American Red Cross
www.redcross.org/services/disaster/keepsafe/
childtrauma.html
Comprehensive resource for childhood trauma.
Free to use.

Trauma Central
http://home.earthlink.net/~hopefull
Extensive "online article" collection links regarding trauma
crisis. User must search links.
Free to use.

Trauma in Pregnancy
eMedicine
www.emedicine.com/med/topic3268.htm
Review of pregnancy and trauma.
Free to use.

The American Association for the Surgery of Trauma
www.aast.org
> Review "Trauma Resources" for injury scoring scales.
> Free to use on this page.

Trauma
eMedicine
www.emedicine.com/med/TRAUMA.htm
> Academic article collection on trauma.
> Free to use.

Disaster and Trauma
Medscape
www.medscape.com/resource/disastertrauma
> Thorough collection of resources.
> Registration required.

Tropical Medicine ✑

USU Tropical Medicine
Uniformed Services University of the Health
Sciences—Bethesda, Maryland
http://tmcr.usuhs.mil
Review "TMCR Diseases."
Free to use.

Division of Parasitic Diseases
Centers for Disease Control and Prevention (CDC)
www.cdc.gov/ncidod/dpd
Thorough review of parasitic diseases.
Free to use.

WHO/TDR Malaria Database
www.wehi.edu.au/MalDB-www/who.html
An information resource for scientists working in malaria
research.
Free to use.

Travelers' Health
Centers for Disease Control and Prevention (CDC)
wwwn.cdc.gov/travel/default.aspx
Comprehensive travel health guide.
Free to use.

The American Journal of Tropical Medicine and Hygiene
www.ajtmh.org/contents-by-date.0.shtml
Academic tropical medicine journal.
Subscription required.

Integrated Consortium on Ticks and Tick-borne Diseases
www.icttd.nl
Search the "Virtual Tick Museum" for an extensive listing of tick literature. User must search links.
Free to use.

Malaria Research and Reference Reagent Resource Center
National Institute of Allergy and Infectious Diseases (NIAID)
www.malaria.mr4.org
Extensive malaria resource.
Free to use.

Tropical Diseases Bulletin
CABI
www.cabi.org/AbstractDatabases.asp?SubjectArea= &PID=82
An abstract database on infectious diseases and public health.
Subscription required.

Malaria Journal
BioMed Central
www.malariajournal.com
Online journal covering malaria.
Free to use.

Filaria Journal
BioMed Central
www.filariajournal.com
> Online journal covering filaria.
> Free to use.

Annals of Tropical Medicine and Parasitology
Maney Publishing
www.maney.co.uk/search?fwaction=show&fwid=142
> Official journal of the Liverpool School of Tropical Medicine
> Subscription required.

Annals of Tropical Paediatrics
Manye Publishing
www.maney.co.uk/search?fwaction=show&fwid=143
> Pediatric health in the tropics and subtropics.
> Subscription required.

Undersea/Hyperbaric ❧

Undersea and Hyperbaric Medical Society
www.uhms.org
> Extensive resources.
> Membership required for selected materials.

Hyperbaric Oxygen Therapy (HBO)
eMedicine
www.emedicine.com/plastic/topic526.htm
> Academic review of hyperbaric oxygen.
> Free to use.

Hyperbaric Medicine Today
www.hbomedtoday.com
> HBO journal.
> Subscription required.

HBO Evidence
The Database of Randomized Controlled Trials
in Hyperbaric Medicine
www.hboevidence.com
> Database for hyperbaric medicine.
> Free to use.

Doc's Diving Medicine
Edmond Kay, MD
University of Washington—Seattle, Washington
http://faculty.washington.edu/ekay

Great diving site.

Free to use.

Bennett and Elliott's Physiology and Medicine
of Diving
Elsevier
http://intl.elsevierhealth.com/catalogue/title.cfm?
ISBN=0702025712

The definitive reference of diving medicine.

Purchase required.

Scubadoc's Diving Medicine Online
http://scuba-doc.com

Comprehensive diving information.

Purchases required.

Urology/Urinary Tract Disorders ∽

Urology, Adult
eMedicine
www.emedicine.com/med/UROLOGY.htm
   Extensive clinical urology article collection reviewing multiple topics.
   Free to use.

Urology
Medscape
www.medscape.com/urology
   Extensive clinical urology resources.
   Registration required.

Urology Notebook
Family Practice Notebook
www.fpnotebook.com/URO.htm
   General medical reference on urology.
   Free to use, but a subscription is available.

Urology
BioMed Central
www.biomedcentral.com/bmcurol
   Online open access journal of urologic disorders.
   Free to use.

The Journal of Urology
Elsevier
www.jurology.com

The official professional journal of the American Urological Association.

Subscription required.

American Urological Association
www.auanet.org

Review "Clinical Guidelines" as a medical resource covering selected topics.

Free to use, but fee required for membership.

Current Opinion in Urology
Lippincott Williams & Wilkins
www.co-urology.com

Professional journal of urological disorders.

Subscription required.

UrologyLinx
www.mdlinx.com/urologylinx/index.cfm

Educational resource for urological disease and news.

Registration required.

Pediatric Urology
eMedicine
www.emedicine.com/ped/UROLOGY.htm

Thorough clinical articles covering urological disorders in childhood.

Free to use.

Weight Loss ❧

Weight Control
Medline Plus
National Library of Medicine (NLM)
www.nlm.nih.gov/medlineplus/weightcontrol.html
> Good selection of weight-control resources.
> Free to use.

Guidelines for Selecting a Weight Loss and
Maintenance Program
American Heart Association (AHA)
www.americanheart.org/presenter.jhtml?identifier=2884
> Fact sheet on weight loss and management.
> Free to use.

Weight-control Information Network (WIN)
National Institute of Diabetes and Digestive
and Kidney Diseases (NIDDK)
National Institutes of Health (NIH)
http://win.niddk.nih.gov/index.htm
> General information on weight loss.
> Free to use.

Obesity and Weight Loss
The National Women's Health Information Center
U.S. Department of Health and Human Services
www.4women.gov/faq/weightloss.htm
  Overview for women on weight loss.
  Free to use.

Weight Loss/Dieting
U.S. Department of Health and Human Services/
National Institutes of Health (NIH)
http://health.nih.gov/result.asp/725
  Multiple weight-loss resources.
  Free to use.

Weight Loss/Obesity
Mayo Clinic
www.mayoclinic.com/health/obesity/DS00314
  Thorough obesity and treatment review.
  Free to use.

Weight Loss: What is Obesity?
The Cleveland Clinic/WebMD
www.webmd.com/diet/what-is-obesity
  Thorough obesity and treatment review.
  Free to use.

Weight Loss Surgery
Medline Plus
National Library of Medicine (NLM)
www.nlm.nih.gov/medlineplus/weightlosssurgery.html
  Thorough resources for weight loss surgery.
  Free to use.

Obesity
The New England Journal of Medicine (NEJM)
http://content.nejm.org/cgi/collection/obesity
Academic collection of obesity articles.

Registration, purchase, or subscription required.

Weight Management/Women's Health
Medscape
www.medscape.com/resource/weightmgmt
Thorough obesity management review.

Registration required.

Wilderness Medicine 〜

Wilderness Medical Society
www.wms.org
> Review "Publications and Resources."
> Membership required; subscription required.

Wilderness Medicine Institute
www.nols.edu/wmi
> "The leader in wilderness medicine."
> Purchase required.

Wilderness and Travel Medicine
eMedicine
www.emedicine.com/emerg/topic838.htm
> General review article.
> Free to use.

Wilderness Emergencies
eMedicine
www.emedicine.com/wild
> Selected topics in wilderness medicine.
> Free to use.

Sirius Wilderness Medicine
www.siriusmed.com
An established leader in Canadian wilderness emergency medical training.
Purchases required.

Wilderness Medical Associates
www.wildmed.com
A world leader in teaching wilderness and rescue medicine.
Purchases required.

Global Medical Rescue Services, Ltd.
www.gmrsltd.com
Offers wilderness and expedition medicine, remote rescue, and survival global training.
Purchases required.

Hypothermia.org
www.hypothermia.org
Useful clinical information on hypothermia.
Free to use.

Wound Care ✑

Worldwide Wounds
www.worldwidewounds.com
    Extensive resource on wound care. See "Links."
    Free to use.

Wound Update
www.woundupdate.com
    Literature review of wound care.
    Free to use, but subscriptions may be required for certain articles.

Wound Care
Advancing the Practice
www.advancingthepractice.org
    Excellent clinical resource.
    Free to use.

Journal of Wound Care
Emap Healthcare Limited
www.journalofwoundcare.com
    Clinical wound-care journal.
    Subscription required.

Wound Healing Society
www.woundheal.org

Professional society.

Free to use, but membership or purchases may be required for certain content.

REFERENCES ✍

Google
www.google.com

Karolinska Institute Stockholm, Sweden
www.mic.ki.se/diseases/index.html

MedWeb
Emory University—Atlanta, Georgia
http://170.140.250.52/MedWeb

Hardin.MD
University of Iowa—Iowa City, Iowa
www.lib.uiowa.edu/hardin/md/index.html

Medical Matrix
www.medmatrix.org/reg/login.asp

MedBioWorld
www.medbioworld.com

Medicine on the Net
HCPro, Inc.
www.hcmarketplace.com/prod-3476.html

Health on the Net Foundation
Geneva, Switzerland
www.hon.ch

Martindale's The "Virtual" Medical Center
www.martindalecenter.com

ASK
www.ask.com